STRONG

IS THE NEW

SKINNY

How to Eat,
Live, and Move
to Maximize
Your Power

JENNIFER COHEN

AND

STACEY COLINO

Harmony Books
New York

Published in the United States by Harmony Books, an imprint of the Crown
Publishing Group, a division of Random House LLC, a Penguin Random
House Company, New York.
www.crownpublishing.com

HARMONY BOOKS is a registered trademark, and the Circle colophon is a
trademark of Random House LLC.

Library of Congress Cataloging-in-Publication Data

Cohen, Jennifer
   Strong is the new skinny : how to eat, live, and move to maximize your
power / Jennifer Cohen and Stacey Colino ; foreword by David Kirchhoff.
       pages cm
1. Physical fitness. 2. Exercise. I. Colino, Stacey. II. Title.
   RA781.C536   2014
   613.7—dc23
                                              2014021072
ISBN 978-0-8041-4051-5
eBook ISBN 978-0-8041-4052-2

Printed in the United States of America

Interior photographs courtesy of Jonah Light
Cover design by Jess Morphew
Cover photograph by Adam Rindy

10 9 8 7 6 5 4 3 2 1

First Edition

I WOULD LIKE TO DEDICATE THIS BOOK TO
MY OVERPROTECTIVE BUT EXTREMELY DEVOTED MOM.
YOU HAVE ALWAYS BEEN MY BIGGEST CHAMPION
AND PARTNER IN CRIME. THANK YOU FOR BEING
THE THELMA TO MY LOUISE.
I LOVE YOU!

ALSO, TO HEATHER JACKSON,
THANK YOU FOR BELIEVING IN ME FROM DAY ONE.
IT HAS MEANT THE WORLD TO ME.
YOU ROCK!

Contents

Foreword

Who am I to write this foreword?

For the better part of fourteen years, I worked for Weight Watchers International, first in helping to start its Internet business in 2000 and later as the CEO of the company. I loved and will always love Weight Watchers. I lost over 40 pounds as a Weight Watchers member, and, in the process, I became a completely different and healthier person. I give myself a lot of credit for ultimately getting there, but I give Weight Watchers even more credit for guiding me.

It means a lot to me that Weight Watchers avoids fad diets, and sticks with proven science and practical insights. They know that the only way to sustainable weight loss and health is by finding a healthy and sustainable lifestyle—and not a crash diet.

This gets me to Jen, Stacey, and this book.

Meeting Jen . . .

Jen had been working closely with Weight Watchers as a key partner in helping us build out our fitness platform when we first met. She partnered with us to produce a series of fitness DVDs, she was a frequent contributor to our website, and she hosted events such as run/walks.

But my first-time meeting Jen was for an interview she conducted with me while writing a review of my book *Weight Loss Boss* for *Forbes* magazine. We immediately hit it off and found ourselves deep in a wide-ranging conversation about nutrition and fitness. I could tell almost immediately that she was a kindred spirit on the crusade to help make a healthier planet.

Since that time, we've stayed in touch and have periodically worked together. One memorable instance was a bit we did together on the show *Extra*. I was promoting my book, and she was promoting her DVDs. It would have been uneventful except for the fact that she demanded that I do exercise demos with her on national TV. Harsh! I was terrified that she would make me do some horribly complicated exercise that would cause me to become a national spectacle. She didn't. This is her magic touch. She's tough, but she always makes her workouts accessible. No embarrassment required. She only demands a willingness to try.

This Book . . .

Fundamentally, what I love about this book is its central message. The point of fitness is getting stronger and healthier. It's about empowerment and doing. This book is *not* about deprivation, suffering, or extremes. Sadly, most diet and fitness regimens are just that. The message of this book is about basking in the energy and good feelings that come from getting stronger.

I love this message because it is the life I've found for myself. I found exercise and, more specifically, resistance training nearly fourteen years ago. I cannot express how it has changed me and made me a happier, more confident, and more energetic person. It is the gift that keeps giving over and over again, and my only hope is that more people will find the same.

Jen and Stacey take their subject matter seriously. They avoid the unproven, and they lean heavily on real science and research, not pipe dreams. Their chapter on nutrition is a true testament to this. You will only find practical wisdom based on sound nutritional science, but delivered in an incredibly straightforward way. The magic of nutrition is not the secret of a peculiar ingredient found in deepest South America, but rather it is in making simple healthy choices a daily part of your life. Jen and Stacey get this instinctively, and they serve up their wisdom on food the way food should be served: simple, well prepared, and with no added junk.

They also get that the secret of good nutrition and physical fitness is as much about your head as it is about your mouth and your muscles. They give proper attention to the importance of getting your head straight, and they offer solid and simple techniques to get your brain in gear. They know that habit creation comes from simple, easy-to-adopt techniques, rather than giant changes. That's more than common sense; it's also based on good research on behavior change. They are giving you state-of-the-art information, but doing it in an incredibly engaging and accessible way.

The heart of this book, however, is in what they know better than most: exercise and the workout. Since I've known Jen, I've always admired her for working tirelessly to make exercise accessible and portable. She believes it should be achievable for anyone, no matter where they are. She requires no gym, and she doesn't believe you should have to spend a million bucks to look like a million bucks. She is a fitness populist.

I read these chapters amazed by the way these two authors found ways of making serious workouts that can be done by anyone, anywhere. In my experience, too many people get intimidated too quickly by working out, and it doesn't have to be that way. You just need good plans. The back half of this book is chock-full of them. Prepare to dog-ear this book into submission.

Indeed, strong is the new (and so much better than) skinny. You don't have to have genetics to get stronger. You don't have to be a certain shape to get stronger. Anyone can and everyone should get stronger. My advice to people over the years on exercise has always been the same:

1. Do it! Believe me when I tell you that a life of fitness will set you free.
2. Don't do it all on day one. Start working yourself into it. Make it fun. Set it to a great playlist. Give yourself a reason to look forward to it.
3. Make it a habit. Find ways to make exercise automatic, not a special event. Book it as an appointment on your calendar if you need to. Set out your gym clothes the night before (my favorite trick!) if that will help.
4. Look for a smart plan that you can grow into. Look for a plan you can start right now, right this second. Look for a plan that you can do in your living room, your backyard, or your hotel room.

For number 4, look no further than this book.

Strong Is the New Skinny is a field manual for a better, stronger, healthier life written by two who know.

Start immediately, don't quit, and never look back.

Cheers,
Dave Kirchhoff

Introduction

We're in the midst of a cultural values shift that's nothing short of awesome: women are no longer interested in starving themselves to become skinny Minnies. Instead, we want to look and feel strong, capable, and empowered. More and more of us want to take full possession of our bodies so we can own them, love them, and nurture them in all the right ways. We want to maximize their potential by building strength, stamina, flexibility, and the sculpted muscles that show what we are truly capable of doing. In short, we want to become our very own badasses, our own superheroes.

Psychologically, our collective ideology of what's attractive has shifted from the damsel in distress to women kicking butt. To going hard or going home. Women's attitudes toward their eating and exercise habits have followed suit: Instead of eating like rabbits or guinea pigs, we're more interested in eating like cheetahs, using food as fuel to power our actions, our movements, our ferocity. Instead of gravitating exclusively toward kinder, gentler yoga and Pilates workouts, women are increasingly turning to hard-core training regimens like Tabata, P90X, Insanity, and CrossFit. In fact, just as Pilates dropped out of the top twenty fitness trends in 2011, boot-camp workouts stepped up in popularity to take its place in health clubs, according to research presented at the 2013 American College of Sports Medicine Health and Fitness Summit.

Consider this: after the 2012 Olympics, a survey by Lifestyle 247 (a company that runs boot camps and fitness retreats in the United Kingdom) found that 72 percent of women would prefer to have a strong, more athletic figure, and 35 percent of women feel "repulsed" by the sight of super-skinny celebrities. On September 30, 2013, *Access Hollywood* declared on its website, "Strong is the new skinny is the fitness mantra of the moment." In December 2013, Reuters ran an article about the changing nature of fitness regimens for women with the headline STRONG IS THE NEW SEXY IN WORKOUTS FOR WOMEN. A consensus is growing that strong is sexy and healthy and hot; striving to be rail-thin is not.

Trust us: we know what we're talking about, because between the two of us, we have lots of experience in this arena. For years, Jen has been a go-to fitness expert for scores of media outlets and celebrity clients, as well as a fitness spokesperson for Weight Watchers International, appearing in two of the company's fitness DVD series and as the host of its popular online "Fit in a Minute" videos. She was one of the featured trainers on the debut season of the TV reality show *Shedding for the Wedding,* where she helped contestants collectively lose hundreds of pounds. She is the health and fitness columnist for Forbes.com and Health.com. Meanwhile, Stacey is an award-winning health and fitness writer as well as a certified Spinning instructor and an Aerobics and Fitness Association of America (AFAA) certified group exercise instructor.

To achieve such get-strong, get-confident goals, it's time for all women to start having a new dialogue with our bodies and start treating, feeding, and moving them in more empowering ways. To get the process rolling, *Strong Is the New Skinny* offers a reality-based diet, lifestyle, and fitness program (the SINS plan, for short) for women who want to crank up their level of health and fitness and become stronger and sexier starting now. It's time to give up the body-bashing and physical faultfinding patterns our culture has encouraged for decades. Instead, the time is ripe to embrace what your body can do, not just how it looks, and find ways to maximize your own physique's strength and power in everyday life.

Indeed, the goal of developing a strong, well-defined body is fast becoming the new inspiration and aspiration in the fitness arena—and for good reason. The reality is that not every woman *can* (or should) be skinny, but every single one of us can be fit, strong, sexy, and healthy. It's a goal every woman should strive for. Why? Because being strong is hot and healthy and vibrant! It's a state that will enable you to achieve your goals in multiple areas of your life and feel good about who you are and what you can do. This book will give you all the tools to become strong from the inside out: nutritionally, physically, psychologically, and emotionally.

That's why your new personal mantra will quickly become *Strong is the new skinny*. The secret to achieving this goal efficiently and effectively is to treat your body like a luxury automobile—by giving it the proper fuel, rest, rejuvenation, and other forms of TLC it needs and deserves and by giving it the right physical challenges. In the case of our bodies, the movement part of the equation means doing the optimal combination of cardio, strength training, and flexibility exercises. Plus, each time you eat nutritious, delicious foods, make sleep and R & R the priority they should be, and get your body moving vigorously, you will be building your self-image and your physical prowess and evolving in the best possible ways. You will be slashing your risk of developing cardiovascular disease, type 2 diabetes, hypertension, breast and colon cancer, osteoporosis, Alzheimer's disease, and many other life-threatening conditions. You also will be treating yourself to increased stamina, a boost in mood, enhanced immune function, and improved concentration, productivity, and memory function. Over time, living a fit and active lifestyle can even help you reverse many of the effects of aging.

Putting these elements together will allow you to stop living a *Groundhog Day* of bad diet and movement choices and negative thoughts—and replace them with positive actions and a take-charge attitude. Taking this approach will help you lose inches, drop pounds, sculpt your body, and feel better about yourself than you ever have. Our goal is to help you enhance and strengthen your physique properly—without causing injury or burnout—and to help you develop the mental vigor you need and deserve to have for life.

But this transformation is not going to happen while you're sitting on your butt (unless you're cycling or lifting weights while you do it). You have to make this pursuit a priority. The reality is that most of us probably don't do everything we want to or think we should do every single day. Our guess is that you find at least a little time to select your clothes, apply your makeup, and style your hair. You might even find time to stop at your favorite java joint and order your preferred pick-me-up on the way to work each day. Are we right? We thought so. But do you make time to do a set of squats or planks or to grill vegetables? Maybe not.

In this book, we're going to help you challenge and push yourself out of your comfort zone so you can get fitter, stronger, and healthier—at your own pace and at any age. When you start seeing yourself progressing and achieving physical feats you didn't think you could, the conversations in your head will begin to change naturally. The critical slumlord will be evicted and replaced by a motivating coach who will convince you that you really can do this and stick to this. This is about building you up, not breaking you down. (*How refreshing,* right?!) This is about finding and harnessing your own internal positive energy so you can reach your potential and become the person you truly want to be. Ultimately, this is about giving your relationship with your body a makeover, one that will help you feel better about yourself from head to toe and inside and out.

Along the way, your self-esteem and self-confidence will soar, and they'll reinforce the good work you've been doing and inspire you to kick it up a notch (or two or three or four if you're already fit and want to train for more extreme challenges).

The great thing about the SINS program's strength-based focus is that the process naturally results in building up your endurance and stamina. Going harder for longer is the key to popular fitness trends like CrossFit and competitions like Tough Mudder and Spartan Races. A person's success in these endeavors is directly proportional to her level of "toughness"—physically, emotionally, and psychologically. The SINS program will build up your toughness; as you gain strength physically, accomplishing tasks that you previously were unable to complete, you also will pump up your confidence and can-do spirit.

As you begin to discover what you are truly capable of physically, mentally, emotionally, socially, and professionally, one aspect of your life will have a positive ripple effect on another. The fitter and stronger you get and the more energy and mental strength and clarity you develop, the more capable you'll feel to tackle other challenges with vigor and confidence. And the better your life will become in the process. We know that's a big promise but think about it: What do you have to lose by trying besides the wicked stepmother or critical slave driver who resides in your head? *Good riddance,* we say.

So think about the shape you want to be in, what you want to achieve, and how you want to feel. Grab the ruby slippers, put them on, then say your goals out loud; repeat them often so you can start to believe in them and achieve them. Believing really does lead to achieving. The truth is that becoming healthy, fit, and strong is about so much more than fitting into your skinny jeans or registering a certain number on the scale. It's about feeling emboldened and empowered and becoming the very best version of yourself that you can possibly be. This is about achieving feel-good, look-good fitness and wellness. Reading and heeding the advice in this book will help you embark on that journey and change your body and your life—for the better. *We promise!*

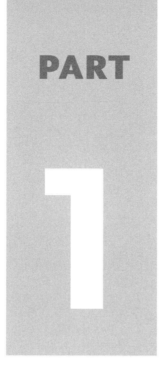

PART

1

INNER STRENGTH

1

Maximizing Your Potential—in Body, Mind, and Spirit

Whether you have a naturally athletic build, a figure that's curvaceous, or one that's willowy, there's good news: you can develop some of the physical attributes you've always wanted but didn't get from Mother Nature or your gene pool. The truth is, with strategic work, every woman can become fitter, stronger, more toned, more self-assured, and sexier. That's an outcome that's realistic and healthy. That's a goal that's achievable and believable. That's a goal that's right for everyone. With the right physical and psychological moves, you really can turn the body you have into the body you want, losing inches, dropping pounds, and developing a stronger, more sculpted look and greater mental fortitude in the process.

If the goal of getting fit and strong has seemed too daunting and complicated in the past, you were probably going about achieving it the wrong way. Sorry to lay that on you, but it's the unvarnished truth. Maximizing your fitness potential isn't as difficult or taxing as many people make it out to be. It involves just three critical elements: a blend of strength-training workouts (a.k.a. resistance training), cardiovascular exercise, and the right moves to enhance flexibility. It really is that simple. Combine these cornerstones of fitness with healthy eating habits—upgrading the nutritional quality of your food choices, using food primarily as fuel, eating regularly, snacking strategically, and exercising "liquid" intelligence (choosing your drinks smartly)—and you'll soon be on your way to a leaner, stronger, fitter physique.

You won't just look better; you'll feel better, too. If you're active enough to break a sweat and get breathless during any given workout, your brain will release endorphins and other feel-good chemicals. Your body will burn fat and extra calories during the session and afterward. Your circulation will improve, and you'll likely get better muscle definition, smoother digestion, and greater strength and stamina for physical activities and the activities of everyday life. By building lean muscle mass through strength training, you'll rev up your metabolism, which will help you burn calories faster and get and stay slim and sculpted for the long haul. Plus, even a brief workout can help regulate your appetite and put the kibosh on your cravings for Girl Scout cookies or other foods you desire. A review of studies published in a 2013 issue of *Sports Medicine* concluded that a single bout of exercise suppresses ghrelin (a hormone that stimulates appetite) while increasing levels of other hormones that inhibit food intake. Really, by exercising regularly, you have nothing to lose except your inertia, lethargy, and body-image blues. So get going already!

The reality is you can work out until you're lobster-red in the face, but if you're eating poorly, it won't make enough of a difference. To see the results you want, it's important to supplement your training with clean eating, which will fuel your body appropriately, while also cutting out unnecessary (and unhealthy) fats, excessive calories, pro-inflammatory foods, and yucky toxins. Get enough sleep, manage stress effectively, and talk kindly to yourself, and you'll make the journey that much easier and more pleasant. These are the essential ingredients that will help you restore, recharge, and refresh your body and mind as you embark on your goal of getting fitter and stronger.

Your body is an incredibly powerful machine—that is, when it's operated and maintained properly. Few things work better the more you use them, but your body will if you take the right steps on a regular basis to restore, recharge, and refresh—the new three Rs. Just as your car needs good-quality gas and oil to run properly, your body needs essential fuels and fluids in the form of clean, anti-inflammatory, health-promoting foods and lots of water. Your body also needs daily breaks for maintenance and recharging: because our bodies are powered wirelessly—we don't have the option of plugging into an external power source—we need to let our internal power source recharge us physically and mentally by getting adequate sleep and rest. The third R—refreshing yourself—can come from resting and relaxing, pampering yourself, giving yourself a well-timed pep talk, and other energy-boosting activities. Taking steps to restore, recharge, and refresh yourself will pay off handsomely as you embark on the *Strong Is the New Skinny* program.

Gaining a stronger, healthier body and mind will help you live life to the fullest, taking on each day with vigor and giving you the confidence to challenge yourself to reach new physical goals. These three assets—getting stronger, living larger, and gaining confidence to challenge yourself further—really do work in tandem. After all, becoming strong and fit is inherently motivating: once you start seeing results, you'll want to keep up the good work to maintain them or to ratchet up your fitness level a notch or two. Feeling fit and empowered can become practically addictive; after you get it, you'll want to do whatever you can to perpetuate that healthy high. When Jen was a trainer on *Shedding for the Wedding,* a reality show where engaged couples who were fairly overweight competed against each other to see who could drop the most pounds, she saw this effect firsthand. Initially, getting the couples to work out hard and cultivate internal discipline and motivation was challenging, even though they all wanted the prize (an all-expenses-paid dream wedding). But, as the participants started seeing their bodies change and felt themselves getting stronger, they became more and more driven and competitive (with themselves and other couples) to see how much fitter, faster, and stronger they could get.

The truth is, a strong, healthy body leads to a strong, healthy spirit and a more inspired, upbeat attitude toward life. *Who wouldn't love that?!* Don't worry, though: you won't have to spend half your life working out in a gym or jogging around a track to get a stronger, slimmer, sexier body. The plan outlined in this book provides a range of multidimensional, compound exercises and workouts that are designed to build strength, stamina, and other aspects of fitness in the most efficient manner possible. You really *can* do this without turning your life upside down. Instead of challenging individual muscles one by one, as many programs do, we combine moves in a way that delivers multiple muscle-strengthening and muscle-sculpting, fat-burning, and body-toning benefits from your neck all the way down to your feet. This is the very best form of multitasking—and it will help you get in the best shape of your life.

The key is to rely on four essential principles of fitness training:

- **Finding the right formula for you.** This involves making the plan personal, then taking ownership of it. Every woman is different in terms of what she likes to do, what she can do, and what she wants to get out of exercise. Before you begin any new venture, it's a good idea to know where you're going or what you're aiming for, don't you think? How can you arrive at your destination if you don't know where (or what) it is? To do that, you'll want to think about how to give your goals our STAR treatment. By that, we mean making them

  Specific with a clear, measurable target so you know what you're working toward;
  Time-based with a set deadline to keep you on track;
  Action-oriented with steps that will help you reach your goal;
  Realistic and achievable for you, given your current level of fitness. If you want to run a 10K race in three months, you might frame your goal this way: Set a **specific** goal (do the race and cross the finish line) and a **time-based** deadline (the date of the race is set, so that's a no-brainer); develop **action-oriented** steps (create stepping-stones such as jogging for 20 to 30 minutes five days a week for the first month, bumping it up to 40 minutes the next month, and increasing your running time to 50 to 60 minutes the third month); and keep it **realistic** (don't aim to achieve a blistering speed during the race if this is your first 10K, or decide to run a marathon instead). If you start with a goal that feels realistic for you to achieve, you'll build confidence that will prepare you for future goals that are more ambitious. You'll learn how to do all this on the pages that follow.

- **Changing up the challenges.** To do this, you'll want to manipulate the lengths and sequences of your workouts, or change the weights you use or the number of repetitions you do on a regular basis. The reality is that sticking with the same old, same old workout routine day after day (a.k.a. exercise monogamy) may seem easy and convenient, but it can lead to exercise monotony, as well as overuse injuries, mental burnout, or a plateau in physiological benefits. It's best to switch up your routine so that you're trying a new cardio activity and fresh strength-training moves every six weeks. This will help keep your workout life interesting and stimulating—and get you better results. It will also help you make continuous progress, without risking injury or boredom. By changing up your workouts, you will challenge different muscle groups, which will force your body to work harder and get stronger.

• **Shocking your body fit.** How? By increasing the intensity of your workouts as your body adapts to each phase. As you get stronger and fitter, you'll notice that the workouts you've been doing have gotten easier. That's a good thing—and a bad thing, too. The good part: It means that you've made lots of progress; it means that what used to be challenging for your body is no big deal now. Congrats on that! The bad part: It means that your muscles, lungs, heart, and other body parts have adapted to the exercises and you are no longer getting as much out of them in terms of cardio-boosting, strength-building, or calorie-burning benefits. This means that you need to take your workouts to the next level, or else you'll end up on an exercise plateau (stuck, in other words).

• **Focusing on neglected muscles.** This involves building strength in an even, systematic fashion so that you can avoid developing muscle imbalances. If you've ever noticed that the right side of your body is stronger than your left (or vice versa) or that certain exercises that require balance are especially challenging, you're personally familiar with muscle imbalances. And you're in good company because we all have them to varying degrees: some people's quadriceps muscles are stronger than their hamstrings; others have an imbalance between the muscles in their abdomen and their back or between their biceps and triceps. (By the way, people tend to focus on building the muscles they can see in the mirror, but it's the ones you don't see that really change your overall physique. That's what we'll be hitting with this plan.) Besides, if you continuously rely on one set of muscles to pick up the slack for another, you can burn out the ones that are doing the most work, which then causes trickle-down stress for adjacent muscles.

By heeding these fitness principles, you'll push your muscles to get fitter, stronger, more flexible and resilient. Strength is yours for the taking. But you will have to work for it, if you want your body to change. With the approach we've outlined, you'll build strength and fitness in a continuous fashion. You'll also avoid falling into the trap of risking acute injuries, overuse injuries, and boredom because you'll be shaking up your routine and the way it makes you feel on a regular basis. By helping you build strength in a systematic, balanced way, you'll also sidestep the problem of developing inequities between different muscle groups.

Bringing Your Head into the Game

Remember, getting stronger isn't just a physical challenge. It also involves an attitude shift and certain changes in your behavior. The desire and drive to change your body and your habits really starts in your head. And the fact is that your mind-set can work with you or against you in this respect. Think about it: would you be more inspired by an upbeat, encouraging coach or a cruel, critical slave driver? We're betting the coach will win this contest. So check in with your thoughts and see which personality they most closely resemble—be honest! As a starting point, consider whether you would ever talk to a friend the way you talk to yourself in your head. If your internal voice belongs to a nasty, negative slave driver, give her the heave-ho and invite a more positive, motivating cheerleader into the picture instead. You can change the conversation that takes place inside your head from one that focuses on your body's deficiencies to one that embraces what's right and what's possible and encourages you to enhance and build on your strengths or natural potential. Making the switch can mean the difference between maintaining the status quo and reaching for and attaining your goals. How you think about and talk to yourself is a choice, and it's one that's within your control.

But getting and keeping the right mind-set also requires training, just as conditioning any other part of your body does. That's because mental fortitude is like a muscle: it needs to be challenged with worthy goals, flexible thinking, and a positive, supportive attitude to grow and develop and get stronger. (You'll learn how to use the right psychological tips and tricks to develop that crucial mental grit and can-do spirit in the pages that follow.) If you haven't pushed yourself in small ways on a regular basis, you may wilt when life gets really challenging. Without mental fortitude, it is nearly impossible to make meaningful or significant changes in your life—like revamping your health habits. To strengthen your mental resolve, it's best to start small by setting attainable goals for yourself: you might vow to eliminate soda from your diet (perhaps by switching to seltzer with a splash of juice, if you like fizzy drinks) or to do 25 burpees or 20 push-ups on a given day, even if you need to take breaks between sets in order to finish them. Once you achieve these small milestones and continue to do them, they'll eventually become second nature to you, and you can then up the ante by setting larger goals, such as working out five times in a week or running six miles without stopping.

The reality is your body and your mind are both much tougher than you think; the key is to tap into their hidden strengths and put them to good use to better the state of your health, your fitness, and your life. The best way to do that is to rely on smart strategies—like exercising first thing in the morning before life's unpredictable nature has a chance to interfere with your good intentions, or stocking your kitchen with wholesome foods rather than junky stuff you tend to eat too much of, or choosing a mantra that inspires you to give the SINS program your best effort—rather than relying exclusively on willpower. This way you'll be setting yourself up to succeed, not fail. Indeed, a recent study from Dartmouth College found that chronic dieters are likely to have greater success if they avoid situations—like viewing lots of desirable foods—that challenge their self-control; the study also found that when perennial dieters overeat, the parts of their brains that balance impulsive behavior and self-control become disrupted, making it harder for them to resist temptation. This isn't surprising given that "willpower, like a muscle, becomes fatigued from overuse," as psychologist Roy Baumeister, PhD, and John Tierney note in their book *Willpower: Rediscovering the Greatest Human Strength,* "but [it] can also be strengthened over the long term through exercise."

Building willpower and mental vigor will help you get stronger on the inside, but this can also help you get stronger on the outside—and the converse is true, too. Getting stronger on the outside can help you feel more empowered, more confident, and more capable. It's a positive ripple effect, a two-way form of synergy between your body and your mind. This book will help you build that bidirectional strength, flexibility, and resilience with challenging physical exercises, a healthy diet, and savvy psychological strategies (learning from your mistakes and your successes, envisioning your optimal performance, finding fitness mentors, and more).

Becoming Your Personal Best

So dare to dream with your eyes open—while you're awake, that is!—and think about the best version of yourself that you can imagine, about who and how you really want to be physically, mentally, and emotionally. Then start your engine and get ready to begin your journey to becoming the strongest, fittest, healthiest, sexiest, most capable version of yourself. To get the party started, you'll want to put on the right headset—the one that makes you feel bold, brave, and powerful—right away. That's what Jen had to do shortly after having a baby in January 2013, and she was asked to shoot a new series of fitness DVDs for Weight Watchers five months later. It was an incredible opportunity (too good to pass up!), but she was still carrying a fair amount of baby weight, and she wasn't in the fittest shape of her life. Rather than caving to the pressure or declining the opportunity, she adopted an attitude that would help her get back into fighting form: First, she pulled out her old fitness DVDs and posted photos of her pre-baby body around her house for motivation. Then, she launched her own version of the SINS program and went back to eating clean, wholesome foods that would help her fuel her workouts and build lean muscle. Most important, she told herself that complaining isn't a valid strategy, but taking action is, and she started acting as if she were already fit (again) until the reality caught up with her mind-set. Relying on these strategies helped her get fit fast—in time for the DVD shoot!

The approach Jen used jibes with research on the powerful connections between what goes on in our bodies and our minds. The truth is that our mind-sets can change the state of our bodies, but our bodies can also change the state of our minds, as social psychologist Amy Cuddy of Harvard Business School notes. For many years, she has been researching the effects of how our body language can influence what's happening in our bodies physiologically as well as our posture and body language. What she has found is that "power posing"—adopting a body posture that conveys competence, power, and confidence—can literally change our feelings, our behavior, and even our hormone levels. Her research has found that adopting a powerful body posture changes our testosterone and cortisol levels in as little as two minutes; she has also found that it increases our appetite for risk, enhances our performance in job interviews, and makes our brains better able to function and cope in stressful situations. That's a whole lot of benefits rolled into a simple change in body posture!

The take-home message: Be willing to take up space in the world by standing tall, looking confident, and fully occupying the space around you, which will make you appear and feel powerful. (By the way, as a bonus, it'll make you look fitter and trimmer, too.) Don't collapse into yourself with poor posture, a weak (or meek-looking) carriage, or fearful facial expressions, all of which can make you look and feel small.

Just as your mind-set can affect your behavior, the converse is true, as well. You can experience a shift in your thinking and your outlook based on your behavior (including your posture) and your feelings. It's a three-step dynamic, really: our mind-sets can change our bodies, the state of our bodies can change the state of our minds, and our behavior can change the results we experience in our lives, as Cuddy puts it. It's not a fluke; research on mood induction, as well as the study of contagious emotions, has found that when people adopt certain facial expressions and body postures, intentionally or not, they can quite literally catch the actual feeling. Here's why: when you model certain facial expressions, postures, or other forms of body language, specific muscle fibers can be activated in your face and body, without your even realizing it, and these tiny muscle movements then trigger the actual feeling by causing the same neurons to fire in your brain as if you were experiencing the feeling naturally.

You can put these principles into play in your get-strong, get-fit plan as well, by acting as if you are already the strong, confident, fit version of yourself that you want to be—until you see the results of your efforts appear naturally. The idea is to fake it until you genuinely feel and believe that you're strong and powerful. Then you can internalize the feeling. So imagine how you'd look, move, and feel if you already had the strong, fit body you've always wanted. Stand tall with an upbeat expression on your face, as if you feel confident and proud. Walk, run, or dance with assurance. Speak with conviction. And dare to go after what you want in life. In other words, start acting as if you're strong, fit, healthy, and super sexy right this minute. Doing this may not get you an Oscar, but it will pump up your belief in yourself, making you feel confident, empowered, and strong. Before you know it, the acting-as-if charade will become a self-fulfilling prophecy—and you'll become the real deal or an even stronger, more capable version of the real deal.

It's time to stop making excuses. We all have them and, yes, some of them are even valid. After all, we're all time starved, stressed, spread too thinly, tired, and yada yada, but getting stronger and fitter will actually help you become more productive, less frazzled, and more capable and energetic, so the effort is time well spent.

If you want to change your habits, you can't just do it by altering your behavior three or four times a week. It has to be a consistent, daily effort so the changes will become ingrained and practically second nature to you, an automatic phenomenon that you don't even have to contemplate. You want to reach the point where you just do these things naturally. Think of making exercise, healthy eating, relaxation, or stretching a daily ritual, just like brushing your teeth, washing your face, or combing your hair. Once you carve out designated time for these endeavors and stick with them, they'll simply become part of the fabric of your daily life.

So the question is, are you in or out? If you want to become stronger, fitter, and healthier, you need to take the plunge and commit. You can't do it halfheartedly. That would be like being a little bit pregnant; you either are or you aren't expecting a baby. Similarly, you either are or aren't going to get fit and strong—it's a choice and a reality, really. If you're ready to embark on this journey, start by banishing words like *can't, should,* and *try* from your vocabulary and replace them with *can* and *will,* as in, "I *can* fit in a workout today" and "I *will* eat five servings of fruits and vegetables daily."

Make this pursuit of strength and fitness a priority, and make time in your schedule to do what it takes. Don't be afraid to test yourself: push through the fear of the unknown and the challenge of moving out of your comfort zone and let yourself come out the other side. You'll be amazed when you discover what you're truly capable of. Ultimately, changing your body and your state of mind and maximizing your assets and your strengths is about reinventing yourself and redefining how you are, both inside and out. As you immerse yourself in the SINS program, you'll start to feel more emboldened, more empowered, and simply more awesome about who you are and what you're capable of. It's a win-win situation.

START A BRAG BOX

There's a lot of talk in the self-help world about the importance of loving ourselves as we pursue new goals. It sounds warm and fuzzy (not to mention kind of touchy-feely). But how exactly are we supposed to do that if the feeling doesn't come naturally?

One key to developing a genuine belief in and appreciation for yourself is to get in the habit of fully experiencing your successes, large and small, and celebrating them. You can do this by recording your progress ("I walked a mile in 14 minutes today—*woo-hoo!*") or your proudest accomplishments in a journal. Or you can start a brag box in which you stash mementos and reminders of your most meaningful successes. Whenever you feel your confidence waning, it helps to peruse your list or to examine the items in your box, to restore your sense of capability and strength.

This will reinforce the great work you've been doing, spur you to keep going, and make you feel proud about what you, your body, and your mind can do.

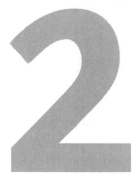

Your Lifestyle Checkup

How well do you really know yourself? Sure, you've been living inside your skin for a long time, so one would assume that you are pretty familiar with yourself (unless you have a serious case of amnesia). But do you really know and understand what makes you tick, what delights you, what empowers you? Be honest. Because if you want to get stronger and fitter, you need to know what you're really like and have a pulse on your strengths and weaknesses—as well as your likes, dislikes, and habits—so you can achieve your goals. If you don't know where you're coming from, how can you possibly tell where you're going? Or whether you've arrived at your desired destination?

That's why it's important to assess where you are now in terms of fitness, diet, and lifestyle. You need to be clear on whether your habits are making you weaker or stronger, as well as what you will need to change to get the results you want. To help you do that, we've created a lifestyle checkup that will help you gauge these elements. Don't worry—the results won't be shared publicly, nor will they go on your report card. This is just a tool for self-discovery, to help you figure out what your patterns have been, where there's room for improvement, and how you can set priorities for making changes that will enhance your ability to get stronger and fitter efficiently. Think of this as the first step in designing a road map that will help you get to a destination of greater strength and fitness. So tell the truth, the whole truth, and nothing but the truth in your responses.

This checkup has two parts. The first measures fitness and nothing but fitness. You'll need to put yourself through your physical paces for this one, so break out your exercise gear and shoes. The main goal behind fitness testing is to get the 411 on your physical condition; that way, you have a benchmark against which you can compare your progress as you embark on the *Strong Is the New Skinny* (SINS) plan. The second part focuses on the rest of your life—your diet, your sleep patterns, and your state of mind. Each of these elements can help or hinder your health and fitness levels.

Let's get started with the helping.

Where Are You Now? Your Personal Fitness Assessment

First, we'll evaluate your cardiovascular conditioning, muscle strength, endurance, and flexibility. Don't stress about your baseline results; the best things about them are that they can help motivate you to launch the fitness program that follows in these pages, and that they give you a yardstick against which you can gauge improvements as you progress through the plan. Record your results, and then retest yourself every four weeks, preferably at the same time of day, to see how far you've come and what your next steps should be.

CARDIO CONDITION. A good way to measure how hard your heart works when you're moving at a steady pace is to do step-ups. (Jog or walk in place for a minute or two.) For this test, you'll need a 12-inch step or platform (in case you're wondering, the stair at the bottom of a staircase typically is too short). As quickly as you can, step up with one foot then the other, and down with one foot then the other in

TOOLS FOR SELF-ASSESSMENT

If you're like many women, you probably weigh yourself fairly regularly. That's a good start, especially if you're trying to manage your weight. If you don't use a scale, that's fine, too. After all, there are other measures that are worth paying attention to—such as your *body mass index* (BMI) and your waist and hip measurements. If you keep a record of these figures, you can better gauge how your body is changing during the fitness program (especially how it's getting leaner and more toned). After all, losing inches of body fat is as important as dropping unwanted pounds.

Let's start with BMI: body mass index is a measure of body fat that's based on your height and weight. To figure out yours, take your height in inches and multiply it by your height in inches. Next, multiply your weight (in pounds) by 703, then divide this number by the previous sum. This number reflects your BMI. Here's what it might mean: a BMI below 18.5 means you're underweight; between 18.5 and 24.9 is normal weight; between 25 and 29.9 is overweight; and 30 and above is obese.

But BMI doesn't tell the whole story when it comes to health and fitness, which is where a tape measure can be useful. Measuring key areas of your body can help you gauge your progress as you work to get stronger. It's essential to measure yourself correctly, though, or you'll get a skewed sense of what's happening with your body. This means don't pull the tape too snugly or let it dig into your skin; also, don't manipulate your body by flexing or tensing your muscles or sucking in your gut while taking your measurements.

Measure yourself naked, ideally first thing in the morning, and hold the tape straight as you wrap it around each area. Measure your bust at the fullest part (when you are naked), usually at the nipple line; your waist at the narrowest part, between your belly button and breastbone; your hips where your butt is fullest; your thighs in the area that has the largest circumference; and your upper arms in the widest part between your shoulder and elbow. Keep a record of these measurements and retake them every two or three months to see how your body is changing as you undertake and stick with the diet and workout program in this book. And if you're done with measuring yourself or trying to measure up to some vague ideal, no sweat; you can gauge your progress on the program in other ways—by noting changes in your strength and stamina, changes in how you move and feel in your body, differences in how your clothes feel and look, and so on. The real value in using these self-assessment tools is that they give you concrete information by which you can measure your progress. Some people like that; some don't. It's your choice as to whether you use them.

a continuous pattern. Do this for 3 minutes. You do *not* need to count your steps. After the 3 minutes are up, measure your heart rate by taking your pulse on your wrist: Extend your left forearm in front of you, with your palm facing up and your elbow slightly bent. Gently place the index and middle fingers of your right hand on the inside of your left wrist, just below the base of your left thumb, until you feel your pulse. Count the beats in 20 seconds then multiply this number by 3 to get your heart beats per minute. Locate your count in the table below.

Age	18–25	26–35	36–45	46–55	56–65	65+
Excellent	< 85	< 88	< 90	< 94	< 95	< 90
Good	85–98	88–99	90–102	94–104	95–104	90–102
Above Average	99–108	100–111	103–110	105–115	105–112	103–115
Average	109–117	112–119	111–118	116–120	113–118	116–122
Below Average	118–126	120–126	119–128	121–129	119–128	123–128
Poor	127–140	127–138	129–140	130–135	129–139	129–134
Very Poor	> 140	> 138	> 140	> 135	> 139	> 134

UPPER-BODY STRENGTH. Doing push-ups is the simplest way to gauge your upper-body strength. So warm up with some jumping jacks or by jogging in place, then get down on your hands and knees, straighten your legs behind you, and place your hands directly beneath your shoulders, palms on the floor. Engage your abs, keeping your body in a straight line, as you lower your body toward the ground, ideally until your elbows are at a right angle; then, push yourself back up to the starting position. Count how many push-ups you can complete in 1 minute. When the time is up, compare your results to the following table to see where you rank within your age group. https://www.presidentschallenge.org/challenge/physical/benchmarks.shtml http://www.topendsports.com/

Age	17–19	20–29	30–39	40–49	50–59	60 +
Excellent	> 35	> 36	> 37	> 31	> 25	> 23
Good	27–35	30–36	30–37	25–31	21–25	19–23
Above Average	21–27	23–29	22–29	18–24	15–20	13–18
Average	11–20	12–22	10–21	8–17	7–14	5–12
Below Average	6–10	7–11	5–9	4–7	3–6	2–4
Poor	2–5	2–6	1–4	1–3	1–2	1
Very Poor	0–1	0–1	0	0	0	0

LOWER-BODY STRENGTH. To measure the strength and endurance of the muscles in your lower body, give yourself the squat test. Stand with your feet hip-width apart, keep your weight over your heels (not the balls of your feet), and squat down until your knees are bent at a 90-degree angle, then lift your body and return to standing. (To make sure you're maintaining good form, you can place a chair behind you and squat down until your butt almost touches the seat before returning to standing.) Count how many squats you can do in 1 minute, then compare your results to the following table.

Age	20–29	30–39	40–49	50–59	60 +
Excellent	> 36	> 32	> 29	> 26	> 23
Good	33–36	29–32	26–29	23–26	20–23
Above Average	29–32	25–28	22–25	19–22	16–19
Average	25–28	21–24	18–21	15–18	12–15
Below Average	21–24	17–20	14–17	11–14	8–11
Poor	17–20	13–16	10–13	7–10	4–7
Very Poor	< 17	< 13	< 10	< 7	< 4

ADVANCED LOWER-BODY STRENGTH. If you're already fairly fit, the one-leg squat is a great way to test your true lower-body strength and your balance at the same time! It also may help identify imbalances between your left and right sides (most people are stronger on one side of their bodies, and that side tends to compensate for the other side while doing regular squats). To do a one-leg squat, stand on your right leg and lift your left foot a few inches off the floor with your left leg extended straight in front of you. Keep your abs tight as you lower your butt toward the floor as if you were going to sit down (you want at least a 45-degree angle on your standing leg), then stand straight up again. Do as many one-leg squats as you can in 1 minute on the right side, then switch to your left side for a minute. Then, compare your results to the following table, based on the number of squats you performed per minute.

Excellent	> 21
Above Average	16–21
Average	10–15
Below Average	8–9
Poor	5–7
Very Poor	< 5

FLEXIBILITY IN THE HAMSTRINGS AND LOWER BACK. Flexibility is an important part of overall fitness, and the sit-and-reach test will help you gauge your status in this area. To do it, remove your shoes and sit on the floor with your legs extended straight out in front of you, your feet about 12 inches apart. Place a yardstick on the floor and put a long piece of masking tape over the 15-inch mark, perpendicular to the yardstick. Place the yardstick between your legs with the 0-inch mark closest to your crotch. With your fingertips in contact with the yardstick, slowly stretch forward with both hands as far as you can go, noting where your fingertips land (to the closest inch). Sit up again then repeat the stretch two more times; record the best measurement, then compare your results to the following table.

	Inches
Excellent	> +11½
Good	+8 to +11½
Above Average	+4½ to +7½
Average	+½ to +4

A BALANCING ACT. Balance is a key component of fitness that can help you avoid injuries in everyday life and when you're working out, so it's worth working to improve yours. To test your balance, stand on your right leg with your right knee slightly bent and bend down to touch your right toes with your left hand, as you raise your left leg behind you a few inches. Return to the starting position without touching down with your left foot. Repeat this as many times as you can in 1 minute, then switch sides and test your left leg's balance. Compare your touches-per-minute results with both legs to the following chart.

Excellent	> 21
Above Average	16–21
Average	10–15
Below Average	8–9
Poor	5–7
Very Poor	< 5

Your Lifestyle Assessment

Read each question or statement carefully, then choose the answer that best describes your attitude or approach to that habit or issue (if two answers apply to you, mark them both and incorporate them in your total tally at the end). Be completely honest! No one else will see your responses, so you're just lying to yourself if you fudge the truth.

1. Which of the following best describes your overall eating habits?
   a)   I eat when I'm hungry and skip meals when I'm not.
   b)   I eat regular meals and snacks on a set schedule throughout the day.
   c)   My eating habits are erratic at best.

2. How many servings of fruits and veggies do you eat on the average day?
   a)   2 to 3
   b)   5 to 7
   c)   1 if I'm lucky

3. When you're facing a difficult challenge—whether it's training for a race, losing weight, or vying for a promotion at work—what kinds of thoughts typically run through your head?
   a)   I experience some self-doubt and try to tolerate it as best I can.
   b)   I try to pump up my confidence by reminding myself of my past successes and that I have what it takes to handle this hurdle.
   c)   I often become critical of myself and get discouraged.

4. How many hours of sleep do you get on a typical night?
   a)   Generally 5 to 6.
   b)   Usually 7 to 9 hours a night.
   c)   It varies widely depending on how busy I am.

5. When choosing what to eat, how do you frame your decisions?
   a)   I have whatever appcals to me at the moment.
   b)   I choose nutritious foods that will fuel my activities.
   c)   I grab whatever is convenient.

6. When your internal voice speaks up in your head—c'mon, we all have one!—who is she most likely to sound like?
   a)   Your mother—sometimes critical, sometimes loving and nurturing
   b)   Your best friend—kind, compassionate, and positive
   c)   Your (fren)enemy—someone who's out to cut you down to size whenever she can

7. How many different colors of foods do you consume from Mother Nature's rainbow (as in, fruits and vegetables) each day?

    a)   2 or 3.

    b)   4 or more.

    c)   1; I like consistency.

8. When you're totally stressed out, what are you most likely to do?

    a)   Call a friend and vent my frustrations.

    b)   Go for a walk or a jog, or meditate.

    c)   Turn to sweet comfort by raiding a coworker's candy dish, the vending machine, or heading to a convenience store for a treat.

9. Which of the following is your primary source of protein?

    a)   Meat or poultry

    b)   A variety of meat, poultry, fish, and/or legumes, nuts, and seeds

    c)   Whatever is quick and accessible

10. How would you describe your snacking style?

    a)   I munch on whatever soothes my jangled nerves—and often eat too much.

    b)   I choose foods that will rejuvenate my energy or satiate my appetite until the next meal.

    c)   I grab whatever is handy.

11. How would you describe your attitude toward exercise?

    a)   I fit it in as often as possible, but blow it off when life gets really hectic.

    b)   Exercise is an essential part of my life; I couldn't survive mentally or physically without it.

    c)   Halfhearted; I work out when I feel like it, not when I don't.

12. Where do most of your dietary fats come from?

    a)   Animal products (meat, dairy, cheese)

    b)   Plant-based foods (including oils—olive, canola, and the like)

    c)   Fried foods (chips, french fries, burgers, etc.)

13. When you experience a setback while pursuing a goal, what are you most likely to do?
    a) Take a break to soothe yourself before deciding whether to try again.
    b) Think about how or where you went wrong and what you can do differently next time.
    c) Give up, thinking you are clearly not cut out for this pursuit.

14. How do you generally feel about your body?
    a) I'm fairly comfortable with it. But I'm definitely aware that there are areas that could be improved upon.
    b) I feel very secure in my own skin and take pride in what my body can do.
    c) I'm unhappy with it. It really doesn't compare well to other women's.

15. Which of the following best describes the way you conduct your life?
    a) I believe that sometimes *good enough* really is good enough.
    b) I generally go hard or go home; I tend to push myself to or past my limits.
    c) I'm a creature of habit and tend to stay within my comfort zone.

SCORING:

Tally up the number of times you chose *a, b,* or *c* as your answer, then read the section that applies most frequently to you. If it's a tie, read both sections; if it's a three-way tie, read all three.

Mostly *a*'s: You've got self-awareness on your side and some good lifestyle habits to go with it. But sometimes you aren't consistent with your eating, sleeping, or exercise patterns, or you don't do what you (probably) know you should be doing when life throws resistance in your path. Try to become more conscious of the daily dietary, exercise, and other health-related choices you make. Also, make a concerted effort to start treating yourself with the TLC and compassion you'd show a close friend; this will make it easier to make and stick with positive changes.

Mostly *b*'s: You are inherently motivated and self-disciplined, and you enjoy pushing yourself physically while also taking good care of yourself mentally and emotionally. Keep up the good work! Just make sure you continue to take time to do things that will restore, recharge, and refresh your body and mind—as well

HOW OLD IS YOUR BODY IN FITNESS YEARS?

It may sound like an odd question but not everyone ages in a linear fashion. You could be forty-five but have the cardiovascular fitness of a twenty-five-year-old—or vice versa. In recent years, researchers at the Norwegian University of Science and Technology in Trondheim, Norway, have developed a way to assess aerobic fitness (outside the laboratory!) and estimate your "fitness age," based on how well your body functions compared to its true biological age.

These researchers have even developed an online calculator (at http://www.ntnu.edu/cerg/vo2max) that lets you see your results immediately. To do the calculations, you'll need to measure your waistline and your resting pulse rate; describe how frequently, long, and hard you exercise; and give your age. You may discover that your fitness age is younger than the number of birthdays you've celebrated, which could inspire you to keep up the great work or even kick it up a notch!

as challenging them in all the right ways. After all, you're aware of your limits, but you don't always honor them. The program that follows will help you with all of this.

Mostly *c*'s: It seems you stick with the familiar (even when it's not working for you) or you feel too overwhelmed to change your habits. Granted, you get points for admitting the truth—and by picking up this book you've already taken the first step toward improving your health and your strength, inside and out. Heed the dietary and fitness advice and the game-changing attitude adjustments that appear on the following pages and you'll be on your way to becoming the stronger, fitter, healthier you you've always wanted to be.

Developing Strength from the Inside Out

Your head can be your friend or foe when it comes to getting stronger, fitter, and sexier. That's because your mind is your most powerful muscle, so you can either flex it to boost your motivation and perseverance (which is great) or clench it to resist your efforts (which is bad). Our advice is to pick option number one. Here's what you stand to gain: a stronger, more consistent sense of motivation, a can-do spirit, a clearer vision of your goals and the mental clarity and fortitude to reach them.

So ask yourself, is your mind your ally or your enemy when it comes to getting fit? When you think about your body—its state, its shape, and its capabilities—do your thoughts sound more like the hip, cool captain of your own cheerleading squad or more like an abusive prison guard? If it's the latter, it's time to evict that critical, sadistic voice and replace it with a more positive one.

The key is to change the way you think and talk about your body; if you don't have anything nice to say, shut up already! Seriously, it's time to reclaim your mind and put it to good use for your body's sake. If you've already got an upbeat outlook, you can kick up your mental strength and positivity a notch or two and take it to the next level. The truth is that you can talk yourself into or out of anything, so why not steer yourself in a positive direction?

After all, your belief system is an important part of getting the results you want. The main difference between a superstar athlete and a regular Jane is that the superstar athlete truly believes she can achieve her goals. She has the confidence, hope, and can-do spirit that will help carry her to the prize (of course, she probably trains like a maniac, too, but it's a mistake to underestimate how big a role mental outlook plays). In fact, research at Santa Clara University in California found that perceived fitness (that is, a person's belief about her level of fitness) is a stronger predictor of the psychological benefits that are associated with exercise than her actual fitness level, as measured by VO_2 max (the maximum rate of oxygen consumption, which reflects aerobic fitness). That's right: believing that you're fit confers more powerful psychological benefits than some measures of actual aerobic fitness. Amazing!

Another body of research suggests that self-efficacy (the strength of your belief in your ability to complete tasks and achieve your goals) helps people adhere to an exercise program better. And some studies indicate that having a sense that you can overcome barriers to physical activity is associated with long-term maintenance of regular exercise. So one of the first steps to achieving a strong, fit body is to strengthen your mind-set. With this chapter, we'll help you build the mental muscle that will enable you to reach your physical goals and develop an arsenal of powerful psychological tools and resources that can help you maximize your potential in all areas.

Plus, cranking up the strength in your head while you're ramping up your physical strength will produce a win-win outcome: the mental vigor you'll be developing will fuel your physical fitness and vice versa, creating an awesome mind-body synergy that will help you grow and thrive and become the best version of yourself yet. After all, when you gain physical confidence, you will likely gain psychological confidence, too. When you condition your body to overcome hurdles or bounce back from setbacks, you will encourage your mind to do the same. It's a two-way street.

It's time, then, to talk yourself into getting fit—or fitter, if you're already fit—starting now. You need to get your head onboard with the plan and condition your state of mind, too. By adopting mojo-boosting mantras, choosing to see yourself in a more flattering light, having mental rehearsals where you visualize your fittest, strongest self in action, and so on, you can build a strong, sexy mind-set from the inside out, one that will help you achieve that reality on the outside, too. There are so many ways to do this. But the first step is to have clear, well-defined goals that outline what you intend to do and how well and often you mean to do it. Spending the time and energy mapping out your goals also sends a signal to your brain that a certain level of commitment, persistence, and ongoing effort will be in order.

The best way to frame your goals is to give them what we call the STAR treatment mentioned earlier:

> **Specific** with a clear, measurable target so you know what you're working toward;
> **Time-based** with a set deadline to keep you on track;
> **Action-oriented** with steps that will help you reach your goal;
> **Realistic** and achievable for you, given your current level of fitness.

To be effective, your goal should be framed in terms of the specific actions you will carry out (which are under your control), not the results you desire (which are outside your control). If your goal is to do a Tough Mudder event, you might state it this way: My goal is to participate in a Tough Mudder in two months; I will get ready by doing the workouts that follow five days per week and by exercising outdoors twice a week. I'll start with 30 minutes and gradually increase the intensity and length of my sessions until I'm ready for race day.

You could even concoct a way to (literally!) see your goals by creating and hanging a storyboard that's filled with images, inspirational quotes, and motivational tips about your goals in your bedroom. Look at your board daily and find a way to design a visual depiction of your progress (with a chart or graph, for example). Having a physical representation of your progress and accomplishments is a good daily motivator to keep up the excellent work.

By using a variety of psychological tips and tricks, you can help yourself gain mental toughness, which can provide a shortcut to lasting self-motivation and progress. Used together, the strategies that follow will help keep you focused and on the fast track to your goal of getting strong and fit—so incorporate as many of them as you can in your life.

THINK ABOUT WHAT'S MOTIVATING YOU. Ask yourself, why do I really want to get stronger and fitter? What's in it for me? Do you want this for intrinsic (internal) reasons (to feel healthy, powerful, and competent) or extrinsic (external) ones (to attract positive attention for your hot-bod-to-be)? The answer matters because research suggests that people who are more intrinsically motivated are often better able to bounce back from disappointing performance and stick with the pursuit of a particular goal because it's personally meaningful. If most of your reasons for embarking on this plan are extrinsic, try to stack the deck in your favor by identifying ways you can better enjoy the process and the feel-good benefits that come from doing so.

PICTURE YOURSELF ROCKING YOUR PERFORMANCE. After Jen watches the movie *Salt* with Angelina Jolie, she visualizes herself as that character—a kickass, strong, superhero of a woman who can tackle anything. Later, she brings that image to mind before her workouts—and ends up feeling as if she can do anything. It's not a fluke: using structured imagery, or visualization, greatly increases "the chance of attaining superior performance because [mental] images program muscles," as sports psychologists Costas Karageorghis and Peter Terry write in their book *Inside Sport Psychology.* The more vivid you can make these images and the more you can recruit each of your senses by imagining the sight, sound, and feel of what you're doing, the more effectively you will prime your muscles for optimal performance when they next engage in that activity.

The reason: "Visualizing yourself performing any skill causes electromyographical (EMG) activity in the relevant muscle groups, similar to what would occur during the physical performance of the imagined movement," as Karageorghis and Terry explain. In other words, these visual rehearsals can actually help improve your physical skills in ways that will enhance your performance.

If you can see it and feel it, you can achieve it.

This is a particularly helpful strategy to use both when you're learning a new skill (and trying to imprint the basic movement pattern in your memory) and when you're trying to refine your skills (and preparing for competition).

DEVELOP A MANTRA. It may sound super spiritual, but a mantra is really just a verbal statement that reinforces a positive mind-set. It can be extremely helpful

Part 1: Save your favorite high-energy songs for a pump-yourself-up playlist. That way, they'll stay fresh, and you won't get tired of them. You can look forward to letting them inspire you to push your pace, your strength, or your intensity when you hear them.

Part 2: Create a playlist that includes words or themes that speak to the intention behind what you're trying to accomplish—songs like "Eye of the Tiger" by Survivor, "Stronger" by Kanye West, "Push It" by Salt-N-Pepa, or "Pump It" by the Black Eyed Peas. Research has found that listening to songs with an emotionally charged message can give you a significant physical and mental boost before engaging in competition or playing a sport.

for keeping your motivation up and your spirits high when embarking on the get-strong program. The key is to come up with a statement that really resonates with you personally, not something generic. It doesn't have to be complicated; it can be something simple like "I'm tough, I'm strong; I can do this!"

Jen's personal mantra is "Believe it; achieve it." Stacey's is "Because I can!"

Start each day by repeating your mantra out loud to get yourself into the right mind-set. Repeat it again throughout the day—including before and during your workouts—to bolster your resolve and inspiration.

Similarly, you can also give yourself verbal cues to enhance your performance during a workout or sporting event. Having a simple phrase in mind—such as "Kick it!" "Pump it up!" "100 percent!" or "Unstoppable!"—can help psych you up to give a full-throttle effort. The more often you give yourself these positive, energizing messages, the more you'll come to believe them.

HUG YOUR FEAR. If the thought of trying a new form of exercise or training for an event that's harder than anything you've done before scares the bejesus out of you, take a breath and then stand up to your fear. If you want to try to get to the bottom of it, you could ask yourself these questions: What's holding me back? What am I really afraid of? Or you may be better off simply acknowledging that you're

PSYCHOLOGICAL STRATEGIES TO SUIT EVERY SITUATION

To develop the mental fortitude you'll want and need to reach your goals with the SINS plan, it's best to rely on psychological strategies that will help you with the situation you're facing. This way, you can personalize the most helpful tips and tricks so they'll suit you and your needs. Here's how:

Situation: You're trying to muster the courage to sign up for a killer boot-camp program you heard about.

Strategies:

Think about what's motivating you.

Hug your fear.

Develop a mantra.

Find a fitness mentor.

Situation: You want to keep yourself energized and driven to see your program all the way through.

Strategies:

Think about what's motivating you.

Develop a mantra.

Re-create a winning feeling.

Find a fitness mentor.

Use pre-workout rituals to put you in the right frame of mind.

Cultivate habits that energize your body and mind.

Situation: You're feeling blah before a workout, and you want to kick up your inspiration a few notches.

Strategies:

Think about what's motivating you.

Re-create a winning feeling.

Picture yourself rocking your performance.

Focus on what's within your control.

Situation: You're in a bad (sad, tense, or otherwise negative) mood, and you just don't feel like working out, even though you know you should suck it up.

Strategies:

Manage your moods.

Make your negative emotions work for you.

Re-create a winning feeling.

Reform the negative chatter in your head.

Situation: You're feeling overwhelmed and intimidated by an intense athletic event that's coming up.

Strategies:

Picture yourself rocking your performance.

Hug your fear.

Focus on what's within your control.

Practice, practice, and practice some more.

Reform the negative chatter in your head.

Situation: You had a dismal workout session yesterday and want to get on a better track today.

Strategies:

Picture yourself rocking your performance.

Anchor yourself to the here and now.

Re-create a winning feeling.

Reform the negative chatter in your head.

Situation: You're in an exercise rut and in danger of falling off the program.

Strategies:

Develop a mantra.

Overcome motivational slumps.

Keep things fresh.

Expect to thrive.

> **Situation:** You rocked at a competition or even in a challenging workout and want to keep that high going.
> **Strategies:**
> Develop a mantra.
> Review what went right.
> Use pre-workout rituals to put you in the right frame of mind.
> Relish your success.

afraid and going for the challenge anyway. When you get to the other side, the fear will be gone, and the payoff (in terms of fitness, confidence, and inner and outer strength) will be enormous. Remember, when you take smart risks, you're likely to get valuable rewards.

MANAGE YOUR MOODS. How many times have you heard that someone bailed on a workout or social plans because she just didn't feel up to or in the mood for it? (Maybe you've even done this yourself.) The reality is that everyone experiences ups and downs. But you don't have to let your training (or the rest of your life) be at the mercy of your moods. Instead, you can learn to regulate your moods with strategies that will help you regain your emotional equilibrium and get the most out of your workouts and your life.

To do this, use relaxation techniques (like doing deep breathing or progressive muscle relaxation exercises or listening to calming music) when you're feeling tense or angry. Take a refreshing shower or a nap or have an energizing snack when you're feeling tired. Bolster your confidence by giving yourself a pep talk when you're feeling stressed out or overwhelmed, and remind yourself that exercise is one of the best mood boosters around. Research has found that it can even alleviate anxiety and depression as well as (and in some cases better than) medications can. And no Rx is required!

FOCUS ON WHAT'S WITHIN YOUR CONTROL. You can't control the weather, other people, or the alignment of the planets, but you can control your attitude toward exercise, competition, and many aspects of your life. Learning to cope with and thrive in the face of adversity and setbacks is a true test of mental toughness. So be prepared (mentally) to deal with unexpected challenges and use flexible strategies to get through, over, or around them. If your workout partner cancels at the last minute, have a backup plan in mind, whether that means going solo or finding a substitute partner. If your hike gets rained out, bring your walk indoors—to a treadmill (set on an incline) at the gym or use a fitness app on your smartphone in your office.

The point is don't get bummed when life throws a wrench in your well-laid plans; get busy coming up with plan B or C by taking steps to control what you can. Complaining isn't a valid strategy. When obstacles get in the way of your fitness regimen, figure out a solution for surmounting them so that you can get to the prize of gaining greater strength, health, and fitness.

ANCHOR YOURSELF TO THE HERE AND NOW. Don't dwell on what happened during yesterday's workout or what could happen tomorrow. Stay focused on the present moment—what you're doing right now! Clear your mind of extraneous thoughts, and if they do float across your consciousness, let them do so without grabbing onto them or reacting to them. Keep your attention and focus firmly squared on what you're doing at any given moment. Aim for total immersion in the experience at hand, and you'll set yourself up for the phenomenon known as "flow," a state of mind in which you become so engrossed in what you're doing that you lose track of time and place as you get in the groove of peak performance. In this state, you feel in control of what you're doing and get pleasure from the experience. It's one of the best ways to get maximum enjoyment and satisfaction out of your training and your life.

OVERCOME MOTIVATIONAL SLUMPS. Believe it or not, one of the best ways to do this is to set small, achievable goals that are based on where you are now—and pursue them with gusto. Reaching these mini milestones will boost your confidence. After all, motivation "is very closely related to confidence because when we believe we can achieve a particular end, we are truly motivated to pursue it with vigor and enthusiasm," as sports psychologists Karageorghis and Terry note. To jump-start motivation when it wanes, it also helps to treat yourself to a change of scenery (perhaps an outdoor workout instead of one at the gym), a new companion (maybe someone you haven't worked out with before), or a different format (perhaps a Spinning or kickboxing class instead of running on the treadmill).

RE-CREATE A WINNING FEELING. Think of a time when you performed at your absolute best, whether it was while playing a sport, giving a presentation at work, or doing something else. Relax and try to remember those feelings of complete confidence, of being fully switched on and in the optimal performance zone. Note what was especially good about your mind-set and your performance and how intensely focused you were. Then try to imagine yourself performing like this again the next time you tackle a workout or another challenge. A friend of ours makes a habit of recalling the "euphoric high"—the sheer thrill—she felt after completing her first marathon and often uses it to kick up her efforts to the next level in her workouts. If you carry a winning mind-set with you, you'll enhance your chances of feeling and functioning at your best.

MAKE YOUR NEGATIVE EMOTIONS WORK FOR YOU. You have two choices: you can either change your perception of your feelings, or you can take action to do something about them. Start by figuring out what's frustrating you. Is it that you're in a fitness rut or you've hit a fitness plateau? If so, you can either change your perception by viewing it as a sign that you've made considerable progress or that you were overly ambitious about the time frame you had in mind, and you need to adjust your expectations. Or you could look at the pattern you've established and tweak something—by doing intervals or changing to a new cardio activity. Either way, that uncomfortable feeling is a signal that some kind of change is warranted.

FIND A FITNESS MENTOR. Look for someone who is more disciplined and fitter than you and try to learn from that person. Ask the person for specific tips to help you along. Steal her best exercise strategies. Let her push and challenge you. Think of her when you suffer a crisis of confidence or motivation. Tell yourself, "If she can do it, so can I!" Having a fitness mentor in your life is like having a hidden stash of effective tools to help you get the job (of getting fit and strong) done, with a little help from your super-fit friend. It's the exercise equivalent of having a business mentor, someone you can emulate, turn to for advice, and learn from at work. Remember, you don't need to reinvent the wheel—in fitness or in life—to find a way to succeed.

KEEP THINGS FRESH. One of the best ways to ward off exercise burnout is to include variety in your workouts—not just variety in terms of the activities and moves you do but also regular changes of venue, the people you work out with, and different sequences in the drills you do. Our close friend Ellen frequently does her strength-training workout in reverse, just to surprise her brain and her body. Even though it's the same workout, just in a different order, she says it feels different to her, which inspires her to work harder. The real benefit to changing up your routine or location regularly is that doing so will help prevent your workouts from feeling stale and help you avoid hitting performance plateaus, both mentally and physically.

REVIEW WHAT WENT RIGHT. After a kick-ass workout or a major accomplishment, take a few moments to recall the different factors that were involved in that peak performance. Use your senses to recall what you saw, heard, or felt during that stellar showing. Try to remember the script that was running through your head and how it may have influenced your performance. There's no guarantee this recipe will lead to the same outcome next time, but there's a good chance that it will. So you'll want to remember it!

USE PRE-WORKOUT RITUALS TO PUT YOU IN THE RIGHT FRAME OF MIND. Having daily rituals can help you stay inspired and focused on what you're doing to move toward your goals. But rituals are highly personal, so it's important to experiment to find what works for you. One woman might get inspired to head to the gym right after her early-morning dog walk. Another might make it a habit to eat a hard-boiled egg with whole-wheat toast before a heavy-duty workout or to wear her favorite exercise clothes or read inspirational quotes to psych herself up for a hard-core session. The specific ideas aren't what matter; what is important is that the ritual you choose motivates you in some way. By consistently using the same psych-yourself-up tactics before a workout or competition, you'll be giving your brain and your body signals that they will need to swing into action and give their best effort very soon.

PRACTICE, PRACTICE—AND PRACTICE SOME MORE. But do it the right way! We're all familiar with the adage that practice makes perfect, but it's only true if the practice is appropriate and gives us valuable feedback that helps us learn. As

Karageorghis and Terry note in *Inside Sport Psychology,* "Inappropriate practice has almost the same effect as no practice or could even result in a decrement in performance." So take your practice sessions seriously, and do your best to master the skills you're trying to develop. Don't sacrifice the quality of your movements for the sake of quantity (as in, reps or the total length of a workout). Focus on executing and fine-tuning the moves, one by one, so that eventually you'll do them correctly without having to think about it. That's the way to practice!

REFORM THE NEGATIVE CHATTER IN YOUR HEAD. It's not enough to silence the negative thoughts that tell you that you aren't fit enough to try kickboxing or Spinning or that you can't hack a cyclo-cross race. A better approach is to replace that naysaying inner voice with one that takes a more productive view; instead of chastising yourself for making a mistake in an athletic event, a more productive approach would be to acknowledge the goof and figure out how you can learn from it. What's the hidden lesson? What could you do differently next time? The idea is to get your inner critic to work for you, not against you, by giving you useful feedback that you can use to help improve your performance. As sports psychologist Shane Murphy, PhD, author of *The Achievement Zone,* notes, "Successful people . . . view mistakes as an opportunity to learn."

Similarly, if you fall off your workout program at any point, shrug it off and simply climb back onboard, without being hard on yourself. Treat yourself with the same kindness and compassion you would show a close friend, and your confidence and self-efficacy will increase. Plus, if you pick yourself up, dust yourself off, and keep moving toward your goal, you can gain wisdom from your errors and bad choices, wisdom that you can then use to benefit yourself in the long run. Susan, a single mother of two, found that despite her best intentions, she frequently missed the afternoon exercise classes she enjoyed at her gym. The unpredictable nature of her work and personal life simply got in the way. Rather than getting mad at herself or frustrated by her life, Susan chose to learn from the pattern: she found a friend who was willing and able to get up 30 minutes earlier in the mornings so they could do pre-sunrise workouts together.

CULTIVATE HABITS THAT ENERGIZE YOUR BODY AND MIND. Building a stronger, fitter body requires consistent energy and effort, so you'll need to replenish your reserves when they start to get low. To some extent, you can do this with your thoughts and feelings, but you'll also want to do this with your lifestyle habits—by regularly getting enough rest and sleep, managing stress effectively, fueling up with healthy foods (see chapter 4), and sustaining a consistently relaxed breathing rhythm.

So ditch the late-night to-do lists and make sleep a priority by carving out ample time for 7 to 9 hours of shut-eye per night. Most of the repair of the body's systems, including our muscles, occurs during sleep, and the brain consolidates new information into memory during sleep. On the other hand, getting too little sleep can take a toll on your workout habits. In fact, a 2012 study by researchers at the University of Chicago found that when healthy adults had their sleep restricted to 5½ hours per night (down from 8½ hours per night), they experienced a 31 percent reduction in physical activity levels and a 24 percent reduction in the intensity of their exercise sessions. This was especially true of people who exercised regularly, which suggests that physically fit people really do need ample sleep to recover from exercise.

Similarly, letting stress get the upper hand can interfere with your efforts to get fitter or pursue other goals. In a recent review of fifty-five studies that examined the influence of stress on physical activity, researchers from Yale University found that both stressful events and the perception of psychological stress consistently have a negative effect on people's efforts to be physically active. (That's a shame because moderate to vigorous exercise can actually relieve stress and boost your ability to cope.)

So make an effort to restore, recharge, and refresh your body and mind on a regular basis by handling these lifestyle habits the right way. Be sure to carve out ample downtime for rest as well as sleep; make an effort to enjoy quiet solitude regularly, even if it's just for 5 to 10 minutes a day, so you can reflect on the goals you're pursuing and recharge your energy and enthusiasm.

RELISH YOUR SUCCESS. Many people make the mistake of reaching for a new fitness goal as soon as they've attained the one they had set their sights on. Whenever you accomplish something you're proud of or you reach a significant milestone in your training, it's important to pause, give yourself a mental high five, and enjoy your success. If you replay it in your mind, you'll reinforce your efforts and your desire to continue to forge ahead in your journey to a stronger, fitter, sexier you. So after completing a 10K race, a team triathlon, a new belt in martial arts, or another meaningful event, take a moment to pat yourself on the back, bask in a bit of pride, and fully appreciate what you've done. You've earned it!

EXPECT TO THRIVE. If you take the right physical steps to get fitter and stronger, and you do whatever you can to prepare mentally, you'll gain trust in your ability to do well in challenging situations. This will help create a self-fulfilling prophecy. If anyone can attest to the truth in this, it's Stacey's friend Nancy, who's on a competitive rowing team. She trains hard with her teammates five days a week, runs on her own once or twice a week, and always looks forward to the regattas. By the time race day rolls around, Nancy has her head in the right place (she expects to work well with her teammates, have a good time, and perform well) because she knows she has worked hard physically to get ready. Thanks to her attitude and work ethic, she trusts the preparation process and expects to thrive from it, and she is rarely disappointed in the outcome of these races. Indeed, if you commit to getting fit and you believe in the training you're doing, you can stop worrying about your performance. Instead, you can let it happen naturally and automatically.

As you strive to achieve your goals, you'll be pushing yourself out of your comfort zone and further into the fit and confident zones, which is where you belong. What's more, you'll set yourself up for a positive ripple effect; feeling fitter, stronger, and more capable in the physical arena can help you start to feel that way in other domains—professionally, socially, emotionally, and so on. Developing this kind of can-do spirit can help you feel more comfortable taking smart risks that could lead to greater fulfillment, empowerment, and self-actualization in your entire life.

Think of it this way: this is your opportunity to live up to your potential and become your best, most authentic self, not the person other people see but the strong, fit person you truly want to be. The process starts in your head, extends to your body, and radiates (positively) into the world from there. So go ahead—set it in motion!

The *Strong Is the New Skinny* Diet Plan

You know the old adage that you are what you eat? Well, it has new meaning when you're trying to build a stronger, healthier body. The truth is, your diet provides the foundation for almost everything your body does, and it's central to any healthy fitness program. It affects whether you gain weight, lose weight, or maintain your current weight. Plus, what you eat provides the fuel for your workouts and the soothing salve for your body's post-exercise recovery. Using nutritious foods as sources of fuel, energy, and vitality will help you build lean, sculpted muscle; a healthy, resilient physique; and an overall sexy body.

Wholesome meals—with the right amounts of lean protein, fruits and veggies, whole grains, and healthy fats—will help you evolve physically and mentally into the kick-ass woman you want to be. But just as important as what you eat is what you don't eat. We know you know where we're going here, but we're going to say it anyway, as it's that important: to become the fittest, hottest you, it's important to eliminate added sugars, refined carbs, processed meats, and unhealthy fats. These items don't offer your body good-quality fuel or sustenance, and they promote sneaky inflammation that can harm your health. So steer clear of them! Plus, if you feed your body junk before exercising, you're unlikely to get the energy, stamina, or strength you were hoping for. Feed your body clean, nutritious food, by contrast, and you'll have plenty of red-hot energy to spare.

Don't worry; the idea here isn't to deprive or starve yourself. That would be torture, and, well, we're just not into that. We're both food lovers! So we make optimal food choices for our bodies—without sacrificing flavor or satisfaction—every chance we get. Think of this as opting for performance-enhancing foods instead of performance-detracting ones, as choosing foods that will restore, rejuvenate, and revitalize you from head to toe. Wholesome, nutritious foods will boost your energy and immune system, help you build and maintain lean muscle mass, promote better digestion and skin appearance, and enhance your brain function and emotional well-being.

To that end, you'll want to choose fresh, whole-plant foods (as in, fruits and vegetables) that represent every color of the rainbow: red, orange, yellow, green, blue, indigo, and violet. (Remember the acronym *ROY G. BIV* that you used as a kid to recall the hues in the rainbow? It applies to the colors of the foods you should be eating, too.) You'll want to choose your complex carbs carefully, as well, opting for whole grains like quinoa, amaranth, oatmeal, and sprouted grain bread, rather than things that are made with worthless white flour. While *carb* has become a four-letter word in recent years—having been blamed for everything from belly fat to fatigue—remember that there are good carbs (like fruits, vegetables, and whole grains) and bad carbs (like simple sugars and processed starches). Carbohydrates provide much of the energy your body needs for exercise and organ function as well as for the metabolism of fat. So it's a huge mistake to eliminate carbs! Just make sure that most of your carbs come from nature, not a box.

In addition, it's important to consume lean proteins, particularly fish, chicken and turkey, lean beef, and lots of legumes (lentils, black beans, chickpeas, and the like). Having adequate protein is critical for building and maintaining muscle mass, for repairing various tissues in the body, and for providing a secondary source of energy for your body (carbohydrates are the main source). It also helps you stay full longer, which can make it a whole lot easier to control your munching and hence your weight. In fact, a 2013 study from the University of Missouri found that having a high-protein snack in the afternoon, three hours after lunch, led to reduced hunger and increased fullness throughout the afternoon.

Also, be sure to opt for healthy monounsaturated and polyunsaturated fats (think olive oil, canola oil, avocado, nuts, and seeds) rather than artery-clogging saturated fats or trans fats. Despite their sometimes negative reputation, fats are important for your health because they transport fat-soluble vitamins, form the major materials of cell membranes and a protective coating for internal organs, and insulate your body against cold temperatures. They also increase the satiety (feelings of fullness) you get from a meal. But as with carbs, there are good fats and bad fats—so, again, choose wisely!

The bottom line: Include moderate amounts of lean protein, healthy fats, and complex carbs in every meal, and you'll keep your appetite in check. You'll be boosting your body's metabolic efficiency simultaneously, so you can build lean muscle mass and burn body fat faster.

Taking this approach will also help you ratchet up your energy and vitality so much that you'll feel turbocharged as you reach for new goals, such as cranking up your strength-training workouts or competing in a challenging athletic event. Achieving these goals essentially requires a back-to-basics style of eating that relies primarily on foods that come from the ground, with moderate portions of meat, fish, and poultry. There isn't a pill on the market that's going to do it for you. While some experts tout the benefits of the latest supplements—such as green coffee-bean extract (which is derived from raw, unroasted coffee beans and purported to have weight-loss benefits), chromium picolinate (a mineral supplement that some people believe can improve blood sugar control and aid with weight loss), and *Garcinia cambogia* (an herbal supplement that comes from the tamarind fruit and supposedly suppresses appetite)—there's little to no evidence that these ingredients boost health or weight management or even that they contain what they claim to. (A recent study by ConsumerLab.com found that most *Garcinia cambogia* supplements don't contain the amounts listed on their labels; one product had only 16 percent of the claimed amount!) If you're inclined to take supplements, ask your doctor about taking a multivitamin and an omega-3 fish oil capsule daily—these have the most evidence in their favor. (Consult ConsumerLab.com to find reputable brands that are free of toxins.)

By sticking with real food, you will get all the essential building blocks you need to construct and maintain a strong, healthy body, along with the nutrients you'll need for optimal energy, wellness, and recovery. Remember, you're in control of what you put in your body, just like you're in charge of which clothes you choose to wear. So make wise dietary decisions. Once you begin to feel and see the difference that comes from smart eating, you'll naturally want to stay on the plan so you can reap further benefits. Feeling strong will give you additional motivation to continue along the *Strong Is the New Skinny* path.

Our dietary plan has three parts that work in a sequential fashion, building upon one another from week to week. The first part, which limits your choices to seven foods in seven days, is designed to help your body reset, allowing you to cleanse your system of junk. At the same time, it will also help you to retrain your taste buds (so they favor healthier foods), get back in touch with your true appetite and satiety levels, fuel up properly for your workouts, shed excess water weight, and gain a greater sense of energy and vitality from your meals. The second and third weeks build upon the first while adding more lean proteins, healthy fats, and complex carbs. The third part—from the fourth week on—continues the building process by allowing you to choose from a broader selection of healthy foods and enjoy good-for-you treats occasionally.

Your Get-Fit, Get-Fierce Plan

Without further ado, let's dive into the details. To help you kick-start your get-fitter, get-fiercer program, the first part of the diet plan calls for sticking with the following seven power foods—the Strong Seven—for the first seven days. These are the latest, greatest superfoods that can help you build muscle mass, torch body fat, and give your body the nutrients it needs for maintenance and repair. By combining protein with carbohydrates and healthy fats in each meal, you'll be able to control your hunger longer, feed your muscles effectively, maintain a more consistent level of energy, and keep your mood and mental performance on an even keel. Pick one food from each pair and incorporate it into multiple meals each day. Here are your choices.

WEEK ONE: THE STRONG SEVEN

Kefir or Greek yogurt. These are great sources of protein and calcium (which are important for building and maintaining muscle and bone mass) and probiotics (which are good bacteria that can promote a healthy digestive system and immune function).

Chia seeds or hemp seeds. They're both rich in omega-3 fatty acids (which have anti-inflammatory and heart-healthy benefits), as well as fiber, protein, iron, magnesium, and potassium. There's a whole lot of nutrition packed into these small seeds.

Tart cherries, blackberries, or raspberries. Besides being low in calories, these vividly colored fruits are great sources of fiber, vitamins A and C, and potassium. Plus, they're loaded with flavonols and polyphenols that offer tremendous antioxidant and anti-inflammatory properties. (Tart cherries contain slightly less sugar and a higher amount of antioxidants than Bing cherries do; blackberries are higher in antioxidants than red raspberries, but red raspberries will suffice if you can't find blackberries.)

Apples or jicama. Both are low in calories and high in fiber, water, and potassium. Apples (especially the peel) also contain quercetin, a health-promoting phytochemical (plant-based pigment) that has antioxidant and anti-inflammatory properties. (Some research suggests that quercetin may even enhance endurance and exercise performance.) Jicama also contains vitamin C, iron, and calcium.

Quinoa or amaranth. These whole grains are high in fiber, antioxidants, and protein, as well as magnesium, potassium, and zinc. Quinoa is also a good source of folate, whereas amaranth boasts impressive amounts of iron and calcium. Consuming these great grains can help stabilize your blood sugar, allowing you to keep your appetite under control and your energy revved.

Wild salmon or lake trout. Besides being protein powerhouses, these cold-water fish are rich sources of omega-3 fatty acids (specifically, docosahexaenoic acid, DHA, and eicosapentaenoic acid, EPA), which combat inflammation and support heart health. They also contain good amounts of niacin, phosphorus, potassium, and vitamins B_{12} and D.

Lentils or edamame. They're both high in protein and fiber, which helps provide a steady flow of energy and assists with appetite control. They're also excellent sources of iron, calcium, potassium, zinc, folate, and vitamin K, which makes them nutritional all-stars.

In addition to these Strong Seven foods, you can eat unlimited amounts of greens—spinach, kale, Swiss chard, bok choy, endive, collard greens, beet greens, mustard greens, turnip greens, kelp, parsley, watercress, and all types of lettuce (red and green leaf, romaine, arugula, mesclun, radicchio, and so on). The more you consume and the more variety you include, the better it will be for you, because you'll fill up for very few calories and get a boatload of nutrients in the process. You can also add as many herbs and spices as you'd like to each meal; not only will this help you vary the flavors and aromas of your meals, but it will also crank up their health-promoting powers because many culinary herbs and spices (such as oregano, rosemary, ginger, thyme, cumin, parsley, and cinnamon) can fight inflammation and pain, stimulate immune function, and promote better digestion, among other health-promoting properties. (Cinnamon can even help with blood-sugar regulation.)

With each meal, as well as between meals, you can drink as much water and white, green, or oolong tea as you'd like. The catechins (a type of phytochemical or plant-based compound) in all teas have antioxidant and anti-inflammatory properties, but white tea has the highest antioxidant content. Tea also may have a mild metabolism-boosting effect that can help you burn calories a bit faster than usual. (But don't add sweeteners to the brew or you'll counteract some of these great effects. Squeeze in a wedge of lemon, instead, if you like its flavor.)

Putting the Strong Sevens into Action

Here are some examples of how you might incorporate these ingredients into your meals.

BREAKFAST: Make a shake with 1 cup of chopped spinach leaves; half a handful of fresh parsley; 1 cup of kefir or Greek yogurt; ½ cup of pitted tart cherries; blackberries, or raspberries; 1 tablespoon of chia or hemp seeds; a dash of coconut water (for extra flavor); and a handful of ice cubes. Blend until it reaches a smooth consistency, then drink up!

SNACK: a cup of tea and an apple

LUNCH: a giant salad with lots of different greens (as much as you'd like), 1 cup of cooked lentils or edamame, 1 cup of chopped apple or jicama, a sprinkling of chia or hemp seeds, and a dressing of olive oil and balsamic vinegar or lemon juice and olive oil

SNACK: a cup of tea and 1 cup of tart cherries or blackberries mixed with 1 cup of plain Greek yogurt or kefir

DINNER: 4 to 6 ounces of baked, broiled, or grilled salmon or lake trout, ½ cup cooked quinoa or amaranth, 1 to 2 cups of kale or Swiss chard sautéed in a tablespoon of olive oil with some chopped or minced garlic

ANOTHER SAMPLE DAY:

BREAKFAST: 1 cup cooked quinoa or amaranth, topped with tart cherries or blackberries and 2 tablespoons of chia or hemp seeds

SNACK: 1 cup of Greek yogurt or kefir

LUNCH: big leafy green salad topped with 4 to 6 ounces of wild salmon or red trout, ½ cup quinoa or amaranth, 1 cup of chopped jicama or apple, and a dressing of olive oil and white balsamic vinegar

SNACK: a cup of tea and ½ cup of tart cherries or blackberries mixed with 1 cup of Greek yogurt or kefir

DINNER: 2 cups lentil soup mixed with 1 cup of sautéed kale or spinach and 1 teaspoon cumin or curry powder; apple slices or jicama spears on the side

WEEKS TWO AND THREE

After the initial kick-start week, you can begin to add (or swap) more fitness-boosting foods, particularly vegetables, fruits, whole grains, and lean proteins. These are all rich in vitamins, minerals, health-promoting phytochemicals, and key macronutrients (such as complex carbs, healthy fats, or protein). Over the second and third weeks, add back one new food per day, keeping your portions under good control. The idea isn't to eat more and more food each day but to add variety to your meals. You could swap a cup of blueberries for one of your daily apples, for example, or have a hard-boiled egg for a snack (or slice it and put it on your lunchtime salad). Or, you could incorporate slices of cucumber, peppers, or carrots into your salad, without eliminating something else, since most nonstarchy veggies are very low in calories.

If you don't have a clue what a true portion of food should be, here's the skinny on what constitutes a proper serving size for various foods:

- 1 cup of raw or cooked vegetables
- 1 whole fruit (such as an orange) or 1 cup of fresh fruit (as in berries or cut-up melon)
- 1 cup cooked beans or legumes
- ½ cup cooked whole grains
- 3 to 4 ounces of cooked seafood, poultry, or lean meats
- 1 cup low-fat or nonfat milk or yogurt
- 1 tablespoon seeds
- ¼ cup nuts

Stick with these serving sizes and your muscles and waistline will thank you! Here's our list of fabulous fitness-boosting foods by category.

Vegetables. They're loaded with vitamins, minerals, and health-promoting phytochemicals, as well as fiber and water. When it comes to vegetables, fresh are best, but the frozen variety is a close second; canned veggies typically contain a substantial amount of sodium, and they're often overprocessed to boot, so use them sparingly and always rinse them (to remove excess sodium) before you use them. These are the best of the bunch:

Acorn squash
Avocado (yes, we know it's really a fruit, but most of us treat it and eat it like a veggie)
Broccoli
Brussels sprouts
Butternut squash
Carrots
Cauliflower
Cucumbers
Eggplant

Green beans
Leeks
Mushrooms
Onions
Peppers (red, green, yellow, orange)
Pumpkin
Sugar snap peas
Sweet potatoes
Tomatoes (see note about avocados)
Zucchini

Fruits. Like veggies, fruits are packed with vitamins, minerals, and health-enhancing phytochemicals, as well as fiber and water, which makes them satiating. In fact, a 2013 study at Purdue University found that when people consumed fruit before a meal, they ate less at the meal that followed; drinking fruit juice didn't have this effect. If it's edible, leave the skin or peel on because the outside layer is a concentrated source of nutrients, especially rich in antioxidants and fiber. Just be sure to wash them thoroughly before eating. Here are some stellar fruit selections:

Apricots	*Oranges*
Bananas	*Papayas*
Blueberries	*Peaches*
Cantaloupe	*Pears*
Grapefruit	*Plums*
Grapes	*Pomegranates*
Honeydew melon	*Raspberries*
Kiwi	*Strawberries*
Mangoes	*Watermelon*
Nectarines	

Legumes. They're loaded with complex carbohydrates, fiber, and protein, a combination that makes them great sources of energy and very filling. In fact, a study from Lund University in Sweden, published in a 2013 issue of *PLOS One*, found that when healthy adults consumed brown beans in their evening meal, they experienced an increase in satiety hormones and a decrease in hunger-promoting hormones (and sensations) the following morning—up to 14 hours later! That's a pretty long-lasting effect. Plus, legumes are rich in vitamins and minerals, and they can easily be added to pump up the volume in many main dishes or salads. Super legume choices include the following:

Black beans	*Great northern beans*
Cannellini beans	*Kidney beans*
Chickpeas (a.k.a. garbanzo beans)	*Pinto beans*

Whole grains. There's a backlash against grains these days, but the truth is muscles need good-quality carbohydrates to supply glycogen for energy, and whole grains are an excellent source of complex carbs, protein, and fiber. They are also packed with various vitamins and minerals, especially antioxidants. Getting strong and fit requires your body to work hard and push its limits; therefore, good-quality carbs (like whole grains) are essential. Thanks to their fiber, they are digested slowly, which boosts satiety, making you feel fuller for longer and assisting with blood-sugar management. No wonder regular consumption of whole grains has been found to help with weight control! A review of fifteen studies on the subject, published in a 2008 issue of *Public Health Nutrition,* concluded that people who have a higher intake of whole grains (about three servings per day) have a lower body mass index and less belly fat than those who consume fewer whole grains. Whole grains are especially important for athletes and very active people, because if these folks don't have enough carbs available for energy, their bodies will start breaking down lean muscle for fuel—a bad, bad outcome! These are great grains to choose from:

Barley	*Rye*
Brown rice	*Sprouted grain bread*
Buckwheat	*Wild rice*
Oatmeal	

Lean protein. There's no doubt about it: protein is essential for manufacturing and maintaining muscle and strength, but you don't have to OD on the stuff. A moderate amount will do. In fact, a 2013 study from Maastricht University in the Netherlands found that while a normal amount of protein—0.8 grams per kilogram of body weight (remember, 1 kilogram equals 2.2 pounds)—helps people lose excess weight, a higher protein intake (1.2 grams per kilogram of body weight) helps them maintain their weight loss after slimming down. The key is to choose lean protein because many forms (like red meat) come with lots of fat. Here are some good choices:

Arctic char	*Buffalo*
Bison	*Chicken breast* (skinless)

Crab	Shrimp
Eggs	Tilapia
Lean beef *(any cut with the*	Tuna *(fresh or albacore)*
words loin *or* round *in it)*	Turkey *(white meat, skinless)*
Mackerel	Wild salmon
Sardines	Yogurt *(the low- or nonfat*
Scallops	*varieties)*

Healthy fats. Dietary fats don't have to clog your arteries. Some can even boost the health of your heart and arteries as well as assisting with the post-exercise muscle repair process, hormonal regulation, satiety from meals, the absorption of certain vitamins, and weight control. The trick is to have the right kinds—as in monounsaturated or polyunsaturated fats and omega-3 fatty acids—in the right amounts (less than 30 percent of your total daily intake). Healthy fat choices include the following:

Canola oil	Nut butters *(such as almond,*
Coconut oil	*peanut, and sunflower*
Flaxseed oil	*seed)*
	Olive oil
	Walnut oil

HERE'S A SAMPLE DAY, USING FOODS FROM WEEKS TWO AND THREE:

BREAKFAST: a cup of oatmeal topped with blueberries, a sprinkling of chia seeds and chopped walnuts; 1 cup Greek yogurt on the side

SNACK: an apple and a cup of tea

LUNCH: a cup of curried lentil soup (with chopped onion, bell pepper, carrots, and kale), served with a broiled chicken breast, lettuce leaves, sliced tomato, avocado slices, and Dijon mustard

SNACK: a small handful of almonds and a pear

DINNER: baked salmon, served over quinoa with spinach sautéed in olive oil, with white bean salad and broccoli on the side; a cup nonfat plain Greek yogurt topped with blackberries for dessert

HERE'S ANOTHER SAMPLE DAY FOR WEEK TWO OR THREE:

BREAKFAST: 2 slices toasted sprouted-grain bread, topped with 2 tablespoons almond butter; 1 cup of blackberries

SNACK: 1 cup of Greek yogurt with blueberries

LUNCH: a cup of black bean soup, and a big salad with lots of greens, cannellini beans, tomatoes, cucumbers, a sprinkling of hemp seeds, and an olive oil–balsamic vinegar dressing

SNACK: I cup of kefir with a nectarine

DINNER: a broiled turkey cutlet; roasted butternut squash, peppers, and green beans

WEEKS FOUR AND BEYOND

Life should be enjoyable, and getting strong doesn't have to mean depriving yourself of edible pleasures. After the third week, you can indulge in a small daily treat if you'd like to—but *small* is the operative word. Mind your portions! Good-for-you choices that won't lead to nosher's remorse include a square or two (as in I or 2 ounces) of dark chocolate; a single-serving box of chocolate milk; a cup of vanilla-flavored almond milk; a glass of red wine; four roasted figs; a cup of baked apple or pear chips; 2 cups of air-popped popcorn; a sugar-free Fudgsicle; a cup of frozen grapes or mango chunks, strawberries, or banana chunks dipped in 2 tablespoons chocolate sauce; or a KIND bar or a Larabar (both are healthy combos of fruits and nuts). Another good option is ½ cup of pistachios. Research from Eastern Illinois University suggests that when people eat pistachios in the shell, they fool themselves into eating less while feeling fuller. Removing the shells and seeing them pile up makes them feel as if they've eaten more than they really have.

HERE'S A SAMPLE MENU FOR A DAY IN WEEK FOUR:

BREAKFAST: a cup of oatmeal topped with roasted apple chunks, a sprinkling of hemp seeds and chopped walnuts, I cup Greek yogurt on the side

SNACK: a pear and a cup of tea

LUNCH: a bowl of white-bean soup, half a sandwich (turkey on rye bread with lettuce, tomato, and mustard), jicama chunks on the side

If you need to slim down in a hurry for a special event, stick with lean proteins and nonstarchy vegetables for a few days. This will help you eliminate water weight quickly and help you look leaner and more taut. Don't do this all the time, though, because your body will get used to it, and you won't see the same results consistently.

HOT TIP

SNACK: a cup of strawberries or banana chunks dipped in 2 tablespoons chocolate sauce

DINNER: baked tilapia served over brown rice with sautéed red pepper, onion, and zucchini strips; 1½ cups blueberries and blackberries for dessert

HERE'S ANOTHER SAMPLE MEAL PLAN FOR WEEK FOUR:

BREAKFAST: Two eggs, scrambled with lots of mushrooms, onions, and spinach; 1 slice toasted sprouted-grain bread

SNACK: apple slices spread with peanut butter and a cup of tea

LUNCH: a large crunchy vegetable salad—chunks of jicama, red pepper, cucumber, carrots, and radishes, on a bed of baby lettuce—topped with canned albacore tuna and an olive oil–balsamic vinegar dressing

SNACK: a cup of low-fat chocolate milk and a banana

DINNER: broiled arctic char served with steamed broccoli and half of a baked sweet potato, a glass of red wine, a cup nonfat plain Greek yogurt topped with mango chunks for dessert

The Calorie Conundrum

In recent years, there's been a lot of debate about whether calories from foods really count or whether certain types of calories are worse for your waistline than others are. The answers are yes and yes! When it comes right down to it, achieving a healthy weight involves getting fit (through exercise) and burning more calories than you consume (from food) each day. So if you end up eating more calories than you burn in your workouts, you're essentially shooting yourself in the foot, sabotaging your weight-management efforts.

But the source of your calories matters, as well. Junk food and sweet treats, for example, tend to be calorie-dense, and they're often metabolized quickly, causing insulin levels to spike, which promotes fat accumulation in the belly. Foods that are loaded with sugar, sodium, and/or fat—all of which are abundant in packaged foods—can also rev up your appetite. Research has shown that these foods can stimulate the pleasure receptors in the brain, just like the addictive drugs heroin and morphine can. So the quality of your calories counts, right along with the quantity.

If you want to count calories, you're welcome to. But you don't have to. If you stick with the recommended portions of different food groups, your total daily calorie count will probably take care of itself. Still, it's smart to become aware of how many calories you generally need per day, based on your height, weight, age, and activity level. That way, you can keep tabs on whether your daily calorie intake is staying in the right slim-down, shape-up, get-strong zone.

The best way to do this is to use the Harris-Benedict equation to calculate your resting metabolic rate (RMR), the number of calories your body needs to simply exist and maintain basic bodily functions like heart rate and breathing. (Math majors, rejoice!) Here's how it works for women:

1. Start with a foundation of 655 calories.
2. Multiply your weight (in pounds) by 4.3.
3. Multiply your height (in inches) by 4.7.
4. Add the totals in lines 1–3 together.
5. Multiply your age by 4.7.
6. Subtract line 5 from line 4: this is your RMR.
7. Factor in your level of physical activity. Multiply the number on line 6 by
    1.2 if you do little to no exercise (if you're sedentary, in other words)
    1.375 if you do light exercise one to three days per week
    1.55 if you exercise moderately three to five days per week
    1.725 if you exercise hard six or seven days per week

The total you end up with reflects the number of calories you need to maintain your current weight. If you want to lose weight at a steady, healthy rate, cut 250 to 500 calories from your daily intake and follow the exercise plan outlined in this book. You'll reach your destination before you know it.

Here's an example of how this might play out in real life—for a woman we'll call Emily, who's thirty-seven and runs or cycles at a vigorous pace for 45 minutes

To avoid letting your body adapt to a certain calorie intake, tinker with the number of calories you consume on a daily basis—by sticking with your usual intake for three days in a row then having a day where you consume enough calories to equal your body weight times 15; then, repeat the pattern. Get those extra calories from protein sources, vegetables, fruits, or starchy carbohydrates (since you'll be keeping your intake of these low the rest of the time). Think of this as a way of tricking your body into keeping a steady metabolic burn going 24/7.

or longer four or five times per week. At 5'9" and 160 pounds, her RMR is in the neighborhood of 1,493:

$$655 + 688 \text{ (160, her weight, } \times 4.3) + 324 \text{ (69, her height in inches, } \times 4.7) - 173.9 \text{ (37} \times 4.7) = 1,493 \text{ RMR}$$

Since she's moderately active, she would need 2,314 calories to maintain her weight (RMR × 1.55). If she wanted to lose weight, she could cut her calorie intake by 250 to 500 calories per day (for a daily intake of 1,814 to 2,064 calories).

Fit Foodisms

If you shift from viewing and treating food as purely a source of pleasure and start looking at it as a source of fuel, you will help yourself build lean, sculpted muscle mass and a healthy, resilient, sexy bod. To do that, you'll want to heed the following strategies, which will help you make the right choices at the right times. We call them "fit foodisms," because they embody sage wisdom that's worth living and eating by.

IF YOU CAN'T KILL IT OR GROW IT, DON'T EAT IT. Real food doesn't have a long shelf life, and nothing good will come from eating lots of processed foods. They're short on nutrients and high on mysterious additives that could do who knows what to your body. Stick with pure, identifiable foods (fruits, vegetables, nuts and seeds, legumes, whole grains, low-fat dairy products, lean meats, poultry, and fish) as much as possible. You don't have to eat them by themselves—you can combine them in dishes or recipes—but it's always good to know what you're actually eating. So when you look at a food label, if there's a long list of ingredients or there are words you don't recognize or can't pronounce, you probably shouldn't be eating it.

CHOW DOWN IN THE MORNING. After sleeping all night, your body and metabolism have settled into resting mode. Having a healthy breakfast—ideally, a combination of complex carbs and protein—will change that by sparking your body's natural calorie-burning power, just like jump-starting an engine does. Plus, you're better off consuming more of your calories in the morning rather than at night, because front-loading your intake will keep you satisfied for longer and give your body the nutrients and calories it needs during the day when you're most active, rather than overloading yourself at night. And starting off with a healthy breakfast sets the tone for the rest of the day, giving you energy (rather than making you feel sluggish as a big plate of pancakes would) and increasing the chances that you'll make better food decisions all day long. But what if you go off the reservation and make some bad food choices? No worries. Everybody does it, and every day offers a chance to start fresh with a healthy breakfast.

EAT REGULARLY. Keep your portions in the reasonable zone, and have a meal or snack every 3 to 5 hours. This will help you avoid the extreme hunger that can cause you to overeat at any occasion where food is present. Plus, if you eat smaller amounts than you're used to throughout the day (including snacks), you'll be able to benefit more often from the metabolic boost you get from digesting, processing, and storing food (a phenomenon called the *thermic effect of eating*). This can help you burn 5 percent more calories per day (an extra 90 calories if you consume 1,800 in total daily). Think of it as a way of continuously stoking your metabolic furnace, as if you were regularly throwing wood on the fire.

ANTI-WATER-WEIGHT FOODS

Certain foods and beverages are natural diuretics. Simply put, consuming them can help flush excess fluids out of your body. Cranberry juice and tea—both the black and green varieties—are well-known for their diuretic properties, but they're not the only beverages or food items that can help your body rid itself of extra fluids. Vegetables like cucumbers, asparagus, celery, fennel, and dandelion greens, as well as herbs such as parsley, coriander, and cardamom, also have natural diuretic effects. In addition, drinking chamomile, alfalfa, or dandelion tea can help you get rid of excess fluids. So can squeezing lemon juice into water, eating a grapefruit, or adding a tablespoon of apple cider vinegar to hot water and drinking this anti-bloat elixir.

Certain minerals—particularly potassium, calcium, and magnesium—can play a critical role in preventing your body from holding on to excess water. It has to do with mineral metabolism and mineral balance—the minerals keep fluids moving properly through your body. If you don't get enough of these essential nutrients from food sources, ask your doctor if you should consider taking a multivitamin and mineral supplement as well as calcium supplements.

REFUEL YOUR BODY PROPERLY AFTER EXERCISING. You've probably heard that you should consume protein right after a weight-based workout to help with muscle recovery and repair. (After all, your muscle fibers experience tiny tears during a strength-training workout.) But that dietary advice misses the mark slightly. What you really want to do is consume a good-quality carbohydrate (such as a banana or orange or whole-grain cereal) to replenish glycogen stores (glycogen is a form of glucose that's stored in the muscles and liver and used as energy for physical activities) immediately after strength-training along with some protein (such as yogurt or low-fat milk); protein helps jump-start the production of glycogen, which is stored in your muscles and used as fuel when you're working out. As nutrition consultant Susan Kleiner, PhD, RD, notes in the latest edition of her book *Power Eating,* "Your muscles are most receptive to producing new glycogen within the first few hours after your workout."

Similarly, it's wise to consume a meal or light snack, consisting of carbohydrate and protein, 1 to 2 hours before exercising to help you power through your workouts without running out of gas. If the timing doesn't work out optimally, at least have something small, like half a banana, 20 to 30 minutes beforehand.

PLAN TO SNACK SMARTLY. Rather than snacking spontaneously, plan your between-meal nibbles ahead of time (in a 200- to 300-calorie portion) so you can avoid the lure of the vending machine or the nearest convenience store when hunger gets a grip on you. The best snacks contain a combination of protein and carbs—such as apple slices with peanut or almond butter or string cheese, baby carrots with hummus, or low-fat plain Greek yogurt with blueberries—real food with real nutrients that will satisfy your hunger, boost your energy, and add some value to your day's nutritional profile. In other words, your between-meal pick-me-ups should contain quality calories that provide a substantial nutritional bang for every bite.

PRIORITIZE PROTEIN. Include a bit of protein in every meal and snack. Why? For one thing, an adequate protein intake is essential for building and maintaining muscle—the stuff you're trying to build. For another, protein takes longer to break down than fats or carbohydrates do, which means you'll feel full and satisfied longer, and have more sustained energy. Plus, if you include some protein in every meal, studies suggest you can burn 5 percent more calories each day.

DRINK LIKE A FISH. We're talking about consuming enough water, not chugging soda, juice, or alcoholic beverages. Water is the most plentiful substance in the body, normally accounting for 60 to 70 percent of your body weight. Your body needs a sufficient water intake to keep your metabolism humming and burning calories efficiently. The US Institute of Medicine recommends that women consume at least 9 cups of fluids per day. Your body may need considerably more than that if you are very physically active. Don't rely on thirst as an indicator of what you need; to stay well hydrated, sip H_2O regularly throughout your waking hours, have a glass of water with every meal and snack, and consume lots of water-rich foods like fresh fruits, vegetables, and soups.

If you don't enjoy drinking water, you can use clever tricks to up your intake—such as training yourself to drink a full glass of water first thing in the morning (put it on your nightstand before you go to bed, as Jennifer does) so you can drink it before you even get out of bed. Also, keep a large bottle, even a pitcher, of H_2O at your desk and make a vow to finish it and refill it before you go to lunch. These are good systems to have in place to create healthier habits. Without these, we wouldn't drink enough water, either!

CONSUME METABOLISM-BOOSTING FOODS. Studies suggest that the EGCG (short for epigallocatechin-3-gallate), a powerful antioxidant that can protect your health, and the caffeine in green tea can rev up metabolism and promote fat burning. Drinking 2 to 3 cups per day seems to confer a 10 to 20 percent boost in your calorie-burning capabilities, an uptick that can last for about 2 hours. Similarly, consuming chili, cayenne, or spicy red pepper can help you burn calories slightly faster, thanks to a compound called capsaicin—the stuff that provides the fiery flavor. In a 2011 study, researchers at Purdue University found that when people added 1 gram (½ teaspoon) of red pepper—a moderate, not overwhelming, amount—to a meal, their appetite was curbed while their energy expenditure increased slightly.

EAT UNTIL YOU'RE SATISFIED, NOT STUFFED. If you take the latter approach (stuffing yourself), it means you're overeating, which won't help you control your weight. Plus, it's harder to exercise when your belly is uncomfortably full because blood flow is being directed toward your digestive system, rather than your muscles. This is one reason why you can get muscle cramps if you eat too much before a workout.

STEER CLEAR OF STOP-SIGN FOODS. Love is a drug . . . and so are pizza, potato chips, and peanut chews. If you have trouble controlling yourself around certain foods, or if some foods are likely to trigger overeating when you're stressed out, for instance, it's best to dodge them entirely or to interact with them only under controlled circumstances. Otherwise, it's like opening Pandora's box. The key is to keep them out of your home—or to indulge only in a situation where limits are built in (like sharing a rich chocolate dessert with a friend at a restaurant).

Getting in the habit of choosing foods that will enhance your energy and fitness levels, rather than simply delighting your taste buds, will help you build the strong, sexy body you've always wanted. So start thinking about your food selections with a "What can you do for me now *and* later?" attitude. This doesn't mean you can't enjoy your meals, but you'll want to start thinking about your food choices as a crossroads where gustatory pleasure and the promise of good health meet. There really is such a place!

PART

2

THE HEAD-TO-TOE

STRENGTHENING

PLAN

5

Back-to-Basic Strength

You may not have thought of it this way before, but your back and shoulders are kind of like the trunk of a tree: they provide the essential support and stabilizing force for the rest of the body that branches off from them. You hear lots of talk in fitness circles about how essential it is to have a strong core because this is where your power comes from, and that's true. But a strong back works in tandem with a strong core; one without the other leaves you lacking in the strength and stability departments.

Having a strong back and shoulders aids you in a variety of everyday moves (from carrying groceries or laundry baskets to lifting young children or luggage) as well as most sports (basketball, boxing, crew, lacrosse, racket sports, soccer, swimming, volleyball, and more). After all, many power moves—pulling, punching, pushing, swinging, throwing, and others—depend on back strength, which gives your body the stability it needs to initiate strong movements from your chest, arms, legs, hips, or core. In fact, the stronger your back muscles are, the more weight-bearing exercises you'll be able to do robustly, safely, and effectively.

In our culture, we talk about the importance of having a strong backbone, meaning the ability to stick with our principles, speak up confidently, stand up for what we believe in, and have the courage to take smart risks. It's a sign of mental vigor, fortitude, and integrity. The same notions can be applied to physical performance, but it's not just the back*bone* that matters here. To develop true physical strength, the muscles in the back—especially the trapezius, rhomboid, latissimus dorsi, and erector spinae muscles—are crucial, too. What people sometimes don't realize is a strong back makes you look super-fit overall. Plus, having a strong back makes you feel more capable and confident. It's a win-win situation.

Gender isn't exactly on our side here. The truth is that women's backs and shoulders generally aren't as strong as men's. Mother Nature compensated for this unfortunate reality by giving us strong hips and legs, but that doesn't help us in the back department. The good news is that this innate disadvantage can be largely eliminated—or at least minimized—with smart strength-training moves.

Many women neglect to work on their backs because, well, they're behind them, and often out of sight means out of mind. Instead, they focus on the body parts they can see in the mirror (the biceps, quads, and abs, for example). That's a mistake because without a strong back, it's difficult to have and maintain good posture, balance, agility, and coordination. Having good posture can make you look thinner and more confident. A strong, toned back and well-defined shoulders will make your waist look smaller (*what woman wouldn't love that?*), which will help you look and be strong, svelte, and sexy. Along with the muscles in your core in the front of your body, your back muscles serve as a corset, providing support and protecting your spine from injury. Without strong back muscles, it's like wearing only half a corset—which really isn't effective! In fact, one of the main reasons people develop back problems is because they have weak back muscles.

The following exercises will help you strengthen, sculpt, and tone the muscles in your upper back and shoulders. A hidden perk: Working on one set of muscles (such as the rotator cuff muscles) often can set you up for developing greater strength in other back muscles (such as the trapezius and rhomboids). It's a positive ripple effect indeed.

In terms of figuring out which dumbbells you should use, here's a good rule of thumb: if you're doing regular strength-training circuits, use weights that are comfortable yet challenging to start. If you can do 8 to 10 reps easily, you should increase the weight. But since the serious benefits come from shocking your body, it's smart to change up the weights you're lifting, too. For example, if you normally

THE TOOLS YOU'LL NEED

The good news is you don't need a whole arsenal of equipment to get a solid workout at home. But you do need a small toolkit with a few key items. (Don't worry; the cumulative cost is much less than a yearly gym membership.) To perform the exercises in this book, you'll need the following:

DUMBBELLS: ideally, a few pairs of weights—including 3 pounds, 5 pounds, 8 pounds, 10 pounds, 12 pounds, even 15 pounds

A STABILITY BALL: the right size for your height—55 centimeters if you're 5'3" or shorter; 65 centimeters if you're 5'4" to 5'10"; 75 centimeters if you're 5'11" or taller

A MAT

RESISTANCE BANDS: a straight one with handles and a circular one

A PLATFORM OR STEP—at least 12 inches

A HEART-RATE MONITOR: to tell if you're maintaining a heart rate in your target zone (65 to 85 percent of your maximum heart rate, for aerobic training)

A STOPWATCH: so you can tell when your time is up for a certain exercise segment in a circuit (or, you can use your smartphone, as Jen does)

A PULL-UP BAR: the kind you can attach to a doorway is optional but highly recommended

A MEDICINE BALL: also optional but recommended

do a set of 15 reps with 8-pound dumbbells, every now and then you could use a heavier weight (say, 12-pound weights) and do 6 to 8 reps instead.

The circuits in this book are based on time rather than reps, so you should mix up your sessions based on the same principles—by starting with a higher weight for a minute (as long as you feel your technique and form aren't being compromised!) to challenge yourself once a week, then dropping down to a lower weight when fatigue sets in. (With this format, you'll want to do as many reps as you can within the time limit.) Remember, your body will adapt fairly quickly to the challenges you're giving it with this program, so try to go with a higher amount

THE PULL-UP DECONSTRUCTED

If you're like most women, doing a pull-up is not part of your exercise repertoire. Whether it's because they're too difficult or you see them as a guy's exercise or there's another reason, it's a shame to shirk pull-ups because they're Jen's favorite exercise of all time. Here's why: they work all of the "pull" muscles in your body—your entire back, your biceps, and your forearms—*and* they're incredible for your abs. Simply put, pull-ups require a lot of muscle groups to work together at once.

Plus, they're a good indication of your level of fitness: anybody who can do a pull-up is in pretty good shape, and anyone who can do 10 or more is clearly in amazing shape. And the truth is that being able to do a set of pull-ups leaves you feeling like a badass in all the best ways!

But let's face it: pull-ups are also hard as hell, especially if you're just getting started. Unlike other exercises that can be completed with just your body weight (like squats, lunges, and push-ups), pull-ups and other exercises that strengthen your pull muscles require at least one piece of equipment (in this case, a bar). On top of all of that, if you can't do one yet, how the heck are you supposed to work up to being able to? It can be an intimidating prospect.

But it can be done if you break the movement down and work up to putting the pieces together. Here's how to learn to do a pull-up:

- Start by doing all the back and shoulder exercises outlined in this chapter—religiously!—for a few weeks. This will help strengthen the muscles you'll need to do a proper pull-up.
- Once you're ready to try a pull-up, start by hanging from the pull-up bar with your feet off the floor, your hands shoulder-width apart, and your palms on the bar (facing away from you). Support your body weight for as long as you can in this position. The next step will be to . . .

- Pull yourself up with your arms until your chin and shoulders are up over the bar, keeping your elbows close to your body. Then, slowly lower yourself to the start position in a controlled fashion. If there's no way you can pull this off, you can place a chair in front of you and put one foot on the seat to give you extra support and leverage during the lift. (Keep in mind that the more you weigh, the more pounds you have to lift in order to complete a pull-up.) Or, you can place a circular resistance band over the bar and tuck the side that's closest to you through the loop and pull it down so it's essentially knotted onto the bar; place one knee—or one foot, if you need more assistance—into the dangling loop for some extra help with the move.

- Modify your hand position to make pull-ups more or less challenging. Having your hands closer together is the easier grip. You can also flip your grip to the underhand style so that your palms are facing you. The wide-apart style, where your palms are facing away from you, is the hardest. All three are truly awesome for the whole upper body.

- Do a set of "jump negative" exercises. This move places the emphasis on the eccentric portion of the movement (the going down part), which will help you improve the quality of your reps. To do these, stand on a stool and place your hands in the proper pull-up position. Skip the concentric part of the movement (the going-up part) and simply jump up to place your chin higher than the bar. As you lower yourself from the bar, do it slowly to a count of 10, trying to resist gravity as much as you can. If you do these properly, you'll hate yourself by the end of one set (6 to 10 reps), but you'll be well on your way to getting stronger!

of weight once a week after you've been on the program for two weeks. You can also go lighter once in a while and power out more reps to surprise your body in another way. With this shock-your-body-fit approach, you'll build toned muscles and get leaner all over. Enough talk—let's get to it!

Back Yourself Up with These Moves

Here's a look at the best exercises for back-to-basic strength.

Push-Up

Lie on your belly with your legs straight behind you and your feet together, the balls of your feet on the floor, and your heels in the air. Place your palms on the floor so they're at chest level and directly under your elbows. Straighten your arms so that your body rises off the floor, keeping your neck straight and your chest lifted, your eyes focused on the floor slightly ahead of you, your abs held tight, and your body as straight as a board. Slowly bend your arms and lower your body toward the floor until your elbows are bent at a 90-degree angle and your upper arms are parallel to the floor; if this is too difficult, lower yourself just halfway down. Exhale then push back up to the starting position.

Plié with Upright Row

Start in a plié position with your feet in a wide stance (slightly more than shoulder-width apart) and your toes pointed out toward the corners of the room. Your knees should be bent slightly, but not to a full 90-degree angle. Hold a dumbbell in each hand with your arms extended in front of you and your palms facing in toward your body. From this position, raise your weights up along the front of your body toward your chest, letting your elbows stick out at your sides (and keeping your shoulders back and down and your chest lifted) as you bring the weights to shoulder level. Lower your dumbbells back to the starting position and repeat. (*Note:* You'll be staying in a plié position the whole time.)

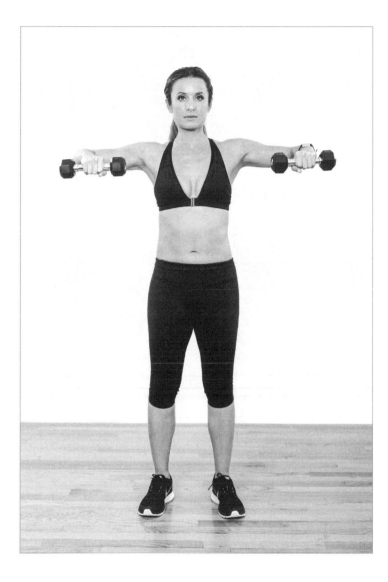

Rotator-Cuff Raise (a.k.a. the Scarecrow)

Stand with your feet hip-width apart and grasp a dumbbell in each hand. Extend your arms out to your sides and then bend them at the elbow into a 90-degree angle with your knuckles facing up toward the ceiling. (You will look like a scarecrow.) Then rotate your forearms down and forward until they are parallel to the ground. The upper part of your arms should remain at a 90-degree angle to your torso at all times. Rotate your weights back up to starting position, and repeat. (By the way, this is a great exercise to get rid of armpit flab.)

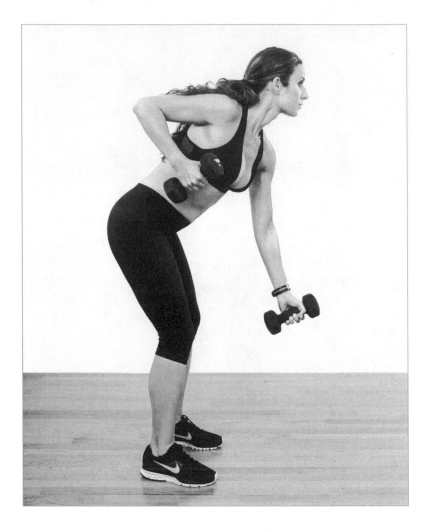

Alternating Big Row

With your feet hip-width apart, hinge forward from your waist so that your torso is leaning over slightly (no more than a 45-degree angle from a standing position). Your knees should be slightly bent. Hold a dumbbell in each hand, your palms facing in toward your body. From here, bend your right elbow and pull your right dumbbell up and back toward your spine, driving from your elbow and keeping it tight against the right side of your body; at the top of the move, the dumbbell will be next to your rib cage. Lower your right arm back to the starting position, then repeat on the left side. Continue this pattern, alternating arms as you work. (For the record, the Dumbbell Row is the same exercise, but both arms move in sync.)

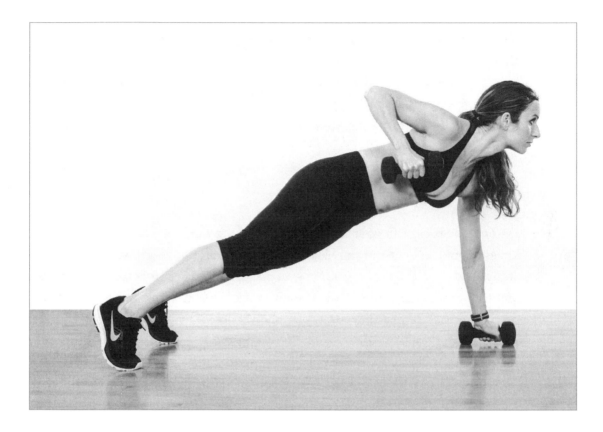

Plank to Row

Get into a push-up position with a dumbbell gripped in each hand (so that the dumbbells are on the ground, rather than placing your palms on the ground). From here, lift your right hand along the side of your rib cage (while holding the dumbbell) and drive your right elbow back and up behind you toward the ceiling, keeping your elbow tight against your body. Lower the weight back to the ground, and repeat on the left side. Continue to alternate sides, keeping your abs tight, your back straight, and your head in line with your spine the whole time.

THE CRANK-IT-UP CHALLENGE: Try adding a push-up between each row.

Superman

Lie on your belly with your feet together, the tops of your feet on the floor and your arms extended straight along the floor above your head. (Your elbows should be next to your ears and your shoulders down.) From here, simultaneously raise your shoulders, your arms, and your legs several inches off the ground. Keep your neck in line with your body and your eyes focused on the floor. Your back will be arched at the top; squeeze your glutes throughout to avoid injury. Hold this position for a moment or two then lower your arms, shoulders, and legs back to the ground. Repeat.

Dumbbell Pullover

Lie on your back with your knees bent, holding a dumbbell in each hand. Your knees should be bent and your feet should be flat on the floor. Extend your arms straight up toward the ceiling above your chest, with your palms facing each other and the weights touching; while keeping your arms straight, move the weights down and back so that they extend beyond the top of your head. As you squeeze your shoulder blades together, bring the weights back toward the ceiling until they are above your chest again. Repeat.

THE CRANK-IT-UP CHALLENGE: Try doing this while lying on a stability ball with your neck and upper body supported, your hips lifted in line with your spine, your knees bent, and your feet flat on the floor; you can also use heavier weights.

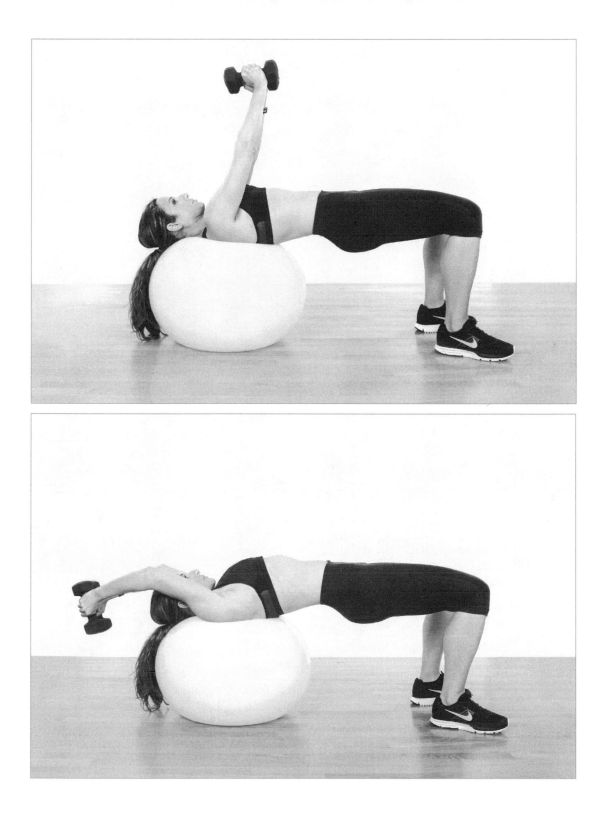

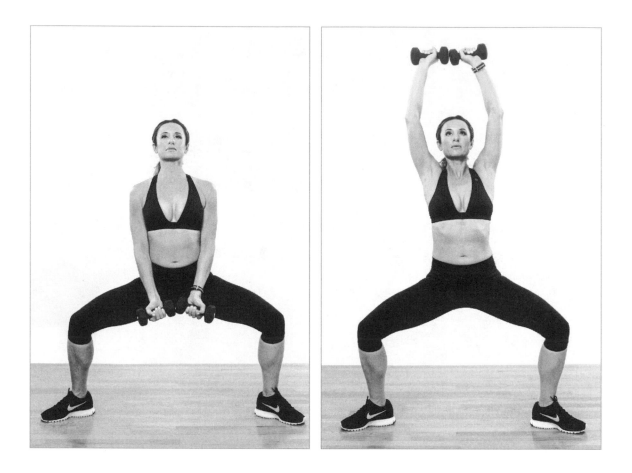

Shoulder Windmill with Plié

Stand in a plié position with your feet in a wide stance (slightly more than shoulder-width apart) and your toes pointed out to the corners of the room. Your knees should be bent as close to a 90-degree angle as possible. Grip a dumbbell in each hand and hold your arms in front of your body with your palms facing front. As you lift the weights out to the sides and overhead in an arc-like movement, they will meet in the middle above your head. Your arms should be fully extended, but there should be a slight bend in your elbows. Make sure your abs are engaged and tucked back toward your spine the whole time. Lower your arms back down to your sides and repeat.

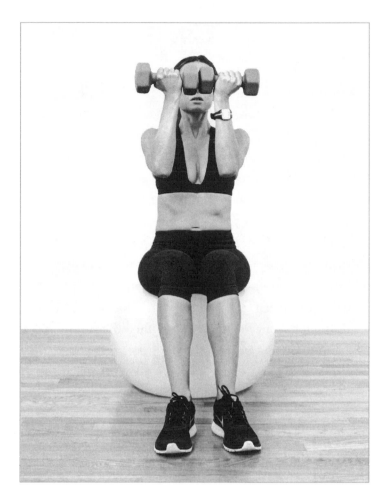

Arnold Press

Sit on a bench or chair, and hold a dumbbell in each hand at chest level with your elbows pointing toward the floor, your palms facing your body, and your knuckles facing the ceiling. To start your press, rotate your elbows out to the sides of your body as you lift your dumbbells up above your head. Your arms should be fully extended at the top (though your elbows can have a slight bend in them); at this point, your palms should be facing forward. Lower the dumbbells back into your starting position, and repeat. Remember to keep your chest up and your back straight with every press.

THE CRANK-IT-UP CHALLENGE: Try doing this move while sitting on a stability ball or use heavier weights.

Inverted Row

You'll need a broom and two stable chairs for this one. Lie on the floor on your back under a low bar that you can reach with your hands when your arms are fully extended. (For a great home-based version of this exercise, you can do inverted rows by lying between two sturdy chairs that have a broom placed across their seats). Your chest should be directly under the bar, and your legs should be extended straight along the ground. Grasp the bar with both hands, slightly farther apart than your shoulders, with your palms facing away from you. As you keep your core tight and your body in a straight line, pull up on the bar, bending your elbows as you raise your body off the ground. (If this is too difficult, you can perform this with your knees bent and your feet flat on the floor until you get strong enough to straighten your legs.) Try to lift your chest all the way up to the bar. When you reach the top, your heels should be the only things still touching the ground. Slowly lower yourself back to the floor, keeping your body in a straight line, and repeat. (*Note:* If you grip the bar with your palms facing you, you'll target your biceps more than your lats; you can alternate between the two styles for added benefits.)

Bent-Over Wide Row

Stand with your feet shoulder-width apart and your knees slightly bent. Hinge forward from your waist while keeping your back flat and your head in line with your spine. Extend your arms straight toward the ground in front of you, holding a dumbbell in each hand. Squeeze your shoulder blades together as you drive your elbows out, up, and back until they reach a 90-degree angle from the sides of your body. (Be sure to keep your abs tucked back toward your spine and your gaze focused on a fixed point on the floor in front of you.) At the top of the move, squeeze your shoulder blades together before lowering your weights back down to their starting position. Repeat.

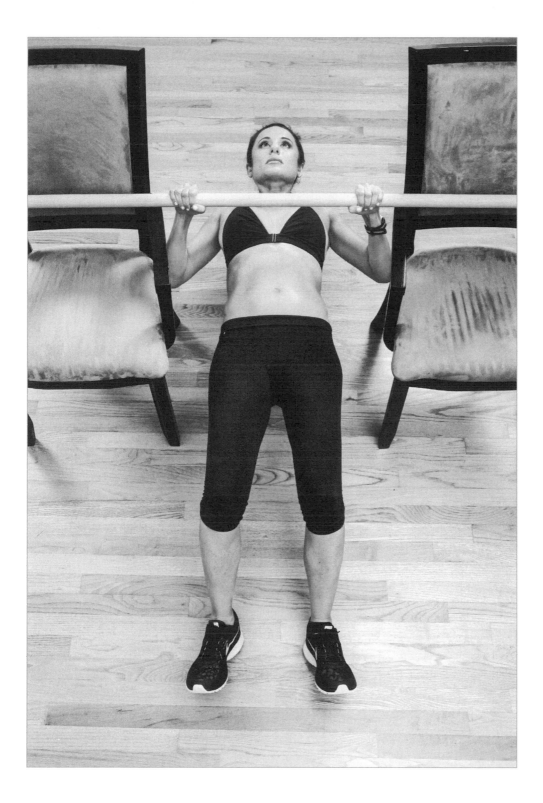

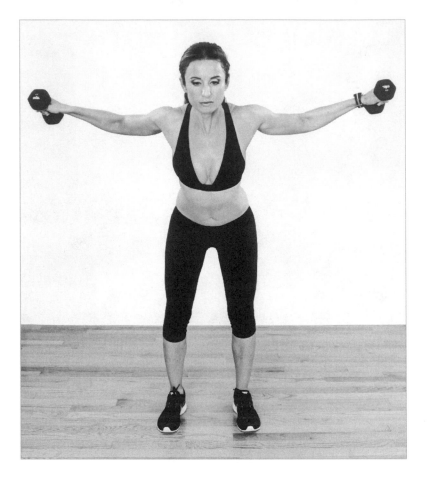

Bent-Over Rear Fly

Stand with your feet shoulder-width apart and your knees slightly bent. Hinge forward from your waist while keeping your back flat and your head in line with your spine. Extend your arms toward the floor in front of you with a dumbbell in each hand, your palms facing each other. From here, lift your arms out to your sides, squeezing your shoulder blades together and keeping your elbows slightly bent. Slowly return them to the starting position and repeat.

THE CRANK-IT-UP CHALLENGE: Step forward into a runner's lunge with one leg, bending your front knee at a 90-degree angle; don't let your front knee extend past your toes, and keep your back heel lifted slightly off the ground. Do rear flies from this position. For an extra challenge, you can also do a whole set with one arm at a time, or a set in which you alternate sides.

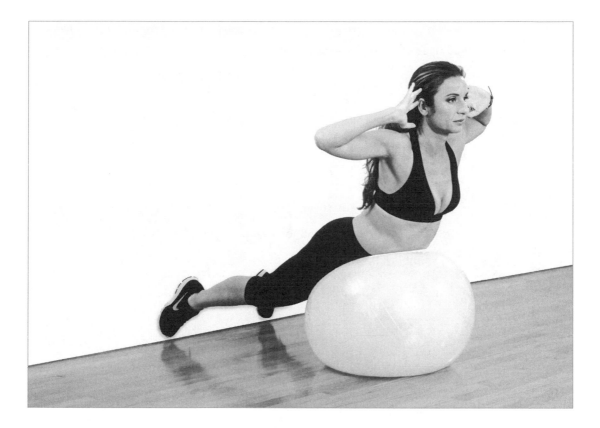

Back Extension on a Ball

Position a stability ball under the front of your hips and lower torso. Keeping your knees straight or slightly bent, place your toes on the floor behind you (or against a wall if you'd like extra stability) and lift your hands behind your head, your elbows extended out to the sides. Slowly roll your body down onto the ball, and then lift your chest off the ball, raising your shoulders until your body is in a straight line from your head to your toes. Repeat. (Make sure your body is in its proper alignment, with your abs engaged and pulled in; don't arch or hyperextend your back.)

Overhead Shoulder Press

Stand with your feet shoulder-width apart and hold a dumbbell in each hand just at shoulder level, with your palms facing forward and your knuckles facing toward the ceiling. Press your arms overhead, and straighten your arms at the top. Return to the starting position and repeat.

THE CRANK-IT-UP CHALLENGE: Try this move while standing on one foot. Switch legs between sets.

Swimmer

Lie on your belly with your arms outstretched overhead, your legs extended along the floor, and your feet together. (Here, too, your elbows should be next to your ears.) Simultaneously raise your head, neck, and shoulders, along with your right arm and your left leg, straight up and off the ground. (To avoid injury, squeeze your glutes and press your pelvic bone into the floor.) At the top of the extension, hold this position for a moment or two, and then release your body back to the ground. Immediately repeat this move on the other side (raising your left arm and right leg along with your head, neck, and shoulders). Continue this pattern, working alternate sides.

6
Armed to Impress

Shapely, sculpted upper arms are among the most prized badges of fitness, a sign that you're truly strong, sexy, and fit. The arms may well be the most viewed body part since they're on display whether you're wearing fitted, tight sleeves; loose, short sleeves; or totally sleeveless styles. One of our friends likes to call stunning, chiseled arms "party arms" because when a woman who has them wears a sleeveless top to a party and reaches for a drink, people—so awed by her guns—often respond with a silent (or softly audible) "ooh!"

But it's more than a matter of aesthetics. Having strong arms is essential for the upper body's pushing and pulling movements, as well as lifting, lowering, and reaching. This is true for everyday activities (like opening jars and hoisting heavy luggage), for contests like Tough Mudders and Spartan Races, and for sports like swimming, tennis, cross-country skiing, boxing, rock climbing, kayaking, and others. Plus, given that we live in such a sedentary culture where we spend hours each day slouched in front of a computer screen or hunched over a steering wheel, having strong arms, along with powerful shoulders and back muscles, helps us maintain the proper range of motion that enables us to carry out the activities of daily living without hurting ourselves.

The good news is your arms will respond relatively quickly to strategic approaches to strength training, especially if you do both pulling and pushing exercises to work all the major muscle groups in different directions. The triceps muscles in the backs of your upper arms are involved in pushing motions; most women use them less often than their biceps, which are located on the fronts of our upper arms and are involved in pulling movements. The best way to get the strong, toned results you want is to do a variety of exercises that target different muscles in your arms and chest (your biceps, triceps, deltoids, and forearm muscles) and to regularly change up the number of sets and reps you do, the amount of resistance you use, and even the angle at which you perform some of the moves.

So if you haven't yet embraced your right to bare powerful arms, it's time to get with the program! Here are the strength-training moves that will help you do just that.

Variations on Push-Ups

The basic push-up was described in the previous chapter. Here are several more challenging variations:

Decline Push-Up

Place your feet on a bench behind you, and then perform a regular push-up. Repeat.

Explosive Push-Up

Assume a plank position and do a regular push-up, making sure to engage your abs and keep your body in a straight line. As you come up, try to push yourself hard so that you lift your hands a few inches off the floor. (If you're worried about landing on your face, it's fine to do these on your knees until you gain confidence.) If you're feeling really strong and confident, try adding a clap in front of your chest while your hands are airborne. As you descend, catch yourself with your hands (and arm muscles, really) and lower yourself into another push-up. Repeat.

Wide Push-Up

Start by lying on your belly, with your feet hip-width apart, your feet flexed, and your toes touching the ground. Place your hands about a foot outside your shoulders on each side with your palms on the ground and your elbows bent. Your fingertips should be facing the sides of the room. Push yourself up into a full plank position with your abs engaged and your body forming a straight line, and then do a series of wide push-ups from this position.

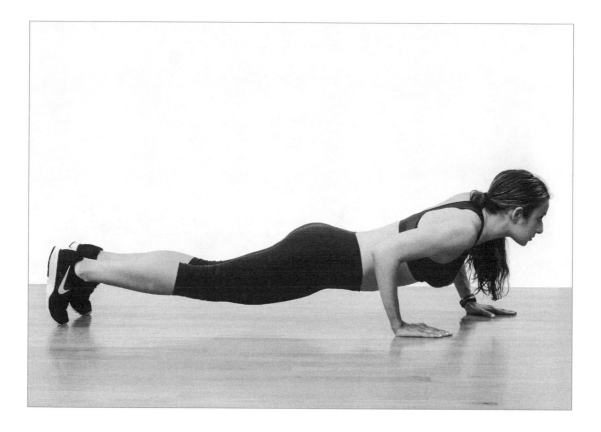

Staggered Push-Up

Start in a regular push-up position but stagger your hands so that one is forward in front of your shoulder and the other is in the usual position. Do half of your reps this way, and then switch your hand positions for your remaining reps.

Close-Grip Push-Up

Start in a regular push-up position but with both of your hands under the center of your chest instead of under your shoulders. Your fingertips should be facing forward. From here, lower yourself into a push-up as far down as you can go. Your elbows will track out to the sides of your body, working your triceps. Push back up and repeat.

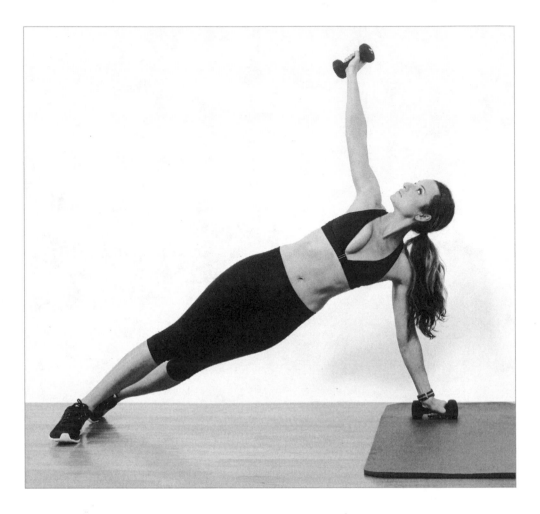

Push-Up to a T

Get into a full plank position. Your weight should be supported by your hands and toes, with your body in a straight line. Do a push-up, keeping your abs pulled in toward your spine. When you come back up to the starting position, transfer your weight to one hand as you rotate your body to reach up toward the ceiling with your other hand. Your body should be in a straight line so you form a T shape. Do another push-up and raise yourself into a T on the other side. Repeat.

THE CRANK-IT-UP CHALLENGE: Do a series of these push-ups with a dumbbell in each hand.

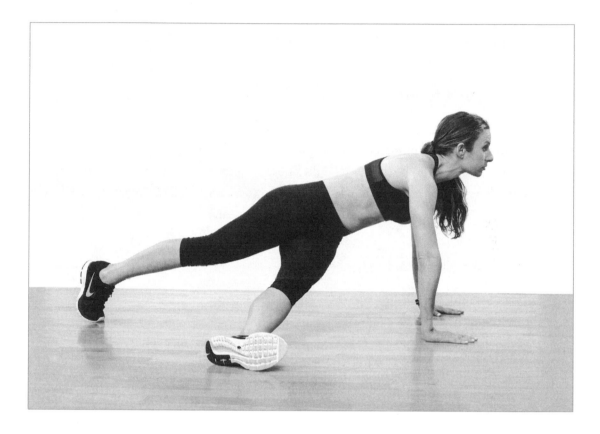

Alternating Cross Leg Push-Up

Start in a regular push-up position. From here lift your right foot and cross your right leg under your body, placing your right foot on the floor to the left of your left foot; do a push-up. Go back to the starting position and then lift your left foot and cross your left leg under your body, placing it on the floor to the right of your right foot; do another push-up. Repeat, alternating legs as you go through your set. (By switching legs as you go, you'll destabilize your body, which further challenges your core and your arm muscles.)

Medicine Ball Push-Up

Do regular push-ups but with one of your hands balancing on a medicine ball; then transfer the ball to your other hand and do another push-up. Continue alternating back and forth, passing the ball.

Walk-Out to Push-Up

Stand tall with your feet hip-width apart. Bend down, place your hands on the floor, and walk yourself out into a plank position. Your abs should be engaged and your body should be in one straight line. Do a push-up. (If you are a beginner, you can do a push-up on your knees.) Once you've completed the push-up, walk your hands back toward your feet and stand up. Repeat.

Side-to-Side Push-Up

Do a regular push-up, and then walk your feet and hands one step to the right while remaining in a plank position. Do another push-up. Move back one step to the left and do a push-up. Repeat, continuing to move from side to side.

Single-Arm Dumbbell Chest Press on a Ball

Lie on your back on a stability ball, with your upper back and neck pressed against the ball. Both feet should be planted firmly on the ground, and your knees should be bent at a 90-degree angle. Hold a dumbbell in each hand and extend your arms toward the ceiling at chest level. While keeping your hips and butt raised, bend your right elbow and lower your right arm until your right elbow is just below chest level. Press the dumbbell up toward the ceiling as you exhale (don't lock your elbow at the top). Repeat until you've done an entire set. After you've completed a full set with the right arm, repeat the work with your left arm. Doing one arm at a time helps to correct strength imbalances in your body. (If you don't have a stability ball, do it on the floor.)

Variations

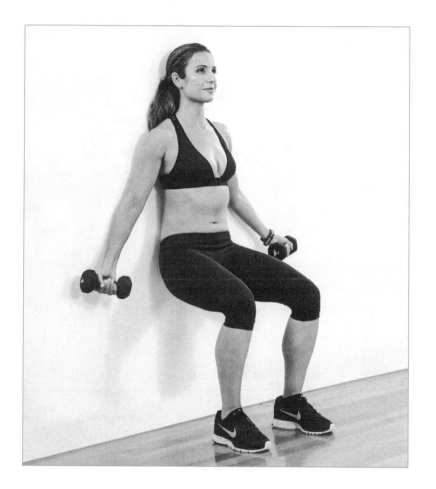

Incline Chest Press in Wall Squat

Stand with your back against a wall with your feet hip-width apart and about 15 to 18 inches away from the wall. Sit into a wall squat with your knees bent as close to a 90-degree angle as possible. Hold a dumbbell in each hand and place your hands out to the sides with your palms facing forward, then bring your arms out in front of you (as if you were going to hug a tree); slowly bring them back to the starting position. (Make sure you're pushing your back into the wall during the entire move.) Repeat.

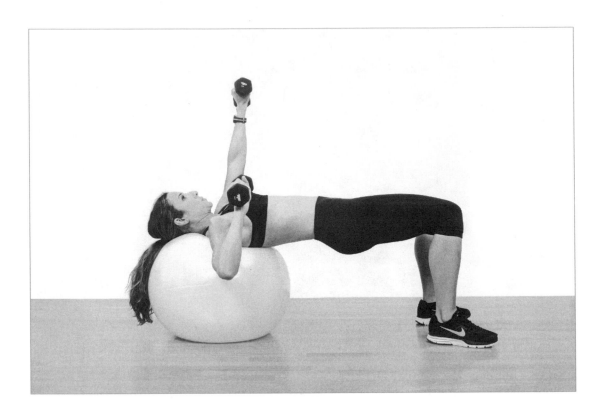

Alternating-Arm Chest Press

Start with both arms extended straight up and then lower one arm; repeat with the other. Keep alternating back and forth while keeping one arm extended straight up.

Chest Press

Lower and raise both arms simultaneously.

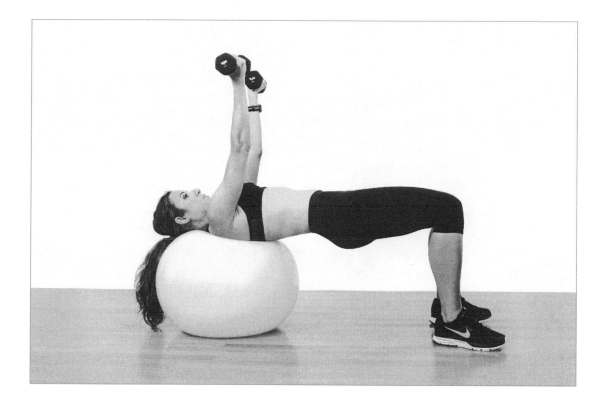

Reverse Dumbbell Press

Lie on your back with your knees bent and your feet flat on the floor. Hold a dumb-bell in each hand with an underhand grip (your palms should be facing you), bend your elbows at a 90-degree angle, and bring the weights just above your chest with your arms straightened but not locked. Then, slowly bend your elbows, lowering the dumbbells down and to your sides until your elbows form a 90-degree angle (keep your elbows in line with your shoulders). Raise the weights to the starting position. Repeat.

THE CRANK-IT-UP CHALLENGE: Try doing reverse dumbbell presses while lying with your neck and upper back on a stability ball; to make it harder, you can also use a slightly heavier dumbbell.

Triceps Dip

Stand with your back to a sturdy bench or chair and bend your knees as if you were going to sit down, but don't! Instead, place your palms on the front edge of the seat about shoulder-width apart. Position your feet in front of you so that your body weight is resting on your arms. Keep your elbows close to your sides and bend your arms, slowly lowering your body until your elbows are bent at a 90-degree angle and your upper arms are parallel to the floor. Your hips should drop straight down toward the ground, staying as close to the seat as possible. Hold the dip for a second, then exhale and straighten your arms back to the starting position. Repeat. (*Note:* Do not lower your body too far down or lean forward as this can overstress your shoulders.)

THE CRANK-IT-UP CHALLENGE: Do triceps dips while elevating your legs on a platform or another chair. Eventually you can also try to do one-handed triceps dips by having one arm extended in front of you while you lift your opposite leg.

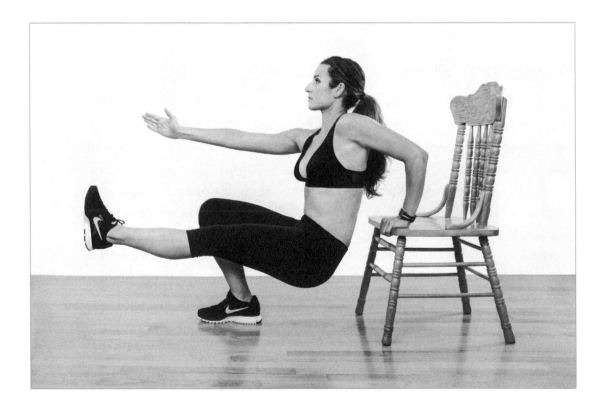

Triceps Tower

Start in a modified plank position on your forearms and toes. Without disturbing your alignment, raise yourself up to a full push-up position on your right hand, then your left hand. Lower yourself back onto your right forearm, then down onto your left forearm. Repeat. Switch the order of sides midway through your reps.

Hammer Curl

Stand with your feet hip-width apart and your arms extended at your sides, your palms facing in toward your body. Grip a dumbbell in each hand and slowly curl the dumbbells up toward your chest by bending your elbows. (Keep your core tight and your elbows locked in by your sides while curling.) Bring the dumbbells as close to your shoulders as you can, then slowly lower them back to the starting position and repeat.

THE CRANK-IT-UP CHALLENGE: To make this move more difficult, try doing hammer curls while you balance on one foot; your other foot should be lifted a couple of inches off the ground. Do a complete set, then switch feet.

In and Out

Stand with your feet shoulder-width apart and your knees slightly bent. Extend your arms straight out in front of you at chest level, holding a dumbbell in each hand. Your palms should be close together and facing each other. From this position, while maintaining a slight bend in your elbows, open your arms straight out to your sides. Keep them at chest level throughout the exercise. Return them to the center and repeat.

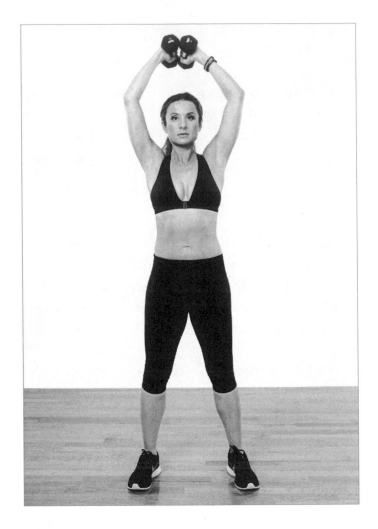

Ballet Arms

Stand with your feet together and hold a light (3-pound) dumbbell in each hand, then gradually work yourself up to 5 pounds, then 8. Start with both arms up above your head, your arms slightly bent at the elbows and your palms facing each other. Keep your core engaged and lower your right arm halfway down to the side to shoulder height. Your arm should remain in the same slightly bent-elbow position. Raise your arm back up, and repeat on the left side.

THE CRANK-IT-UP CHALLENGE: Add a lateral side-to-side squat by stepping out on the same side as the arm that is lowering the weight, into a 90-degree squat. (Or if you want to channel your inner ballerina, plié instead.)

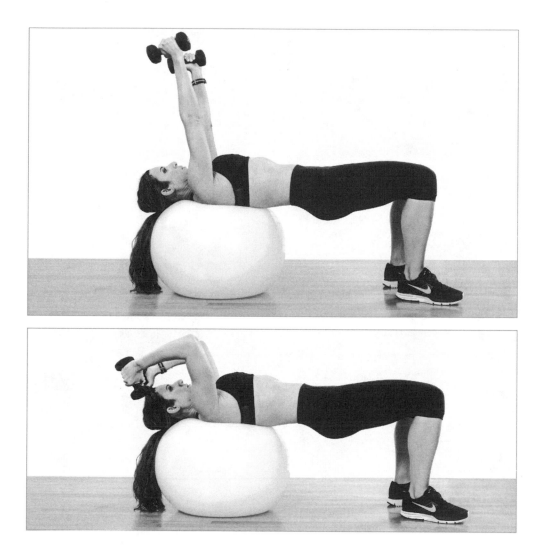

Skull Crusher on a Stability Ball

Lie with your upper back and neck on the ball and both legs planted firmly on the ground, with your knees bent at a 90-degree angle; your torso should be parallel to the floor. Hold a dumbbell in each hand and extend your arms straight up above your head. From this position, keeping a firm grasp on the weights, lower the dumbbells toward your forehead by bending your elbows at a 90-degree angle. Then raise the dumbbells back up to the extended position. Repeat.

VARIATION: If you are a beginner or don't have an exercise ball handy, try doing these on a weight bench or on the floor first.

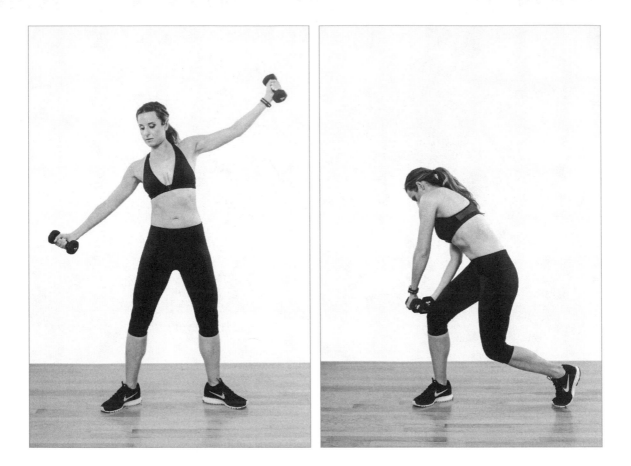

Grapple Throw

Stand with your feet shoulder-width apart, holding a dumbbell in each hand next to your right hip. With your arms slightly bent and your abs engaged, lift the dumbbells up and over your head until you reach your other hip in a circular motion. Reverse the motion and return the weights to the right side; continue doing this back and forth (going in each direction constitutes a rep). (*Note:* This exercise works your core as well as your arms.)

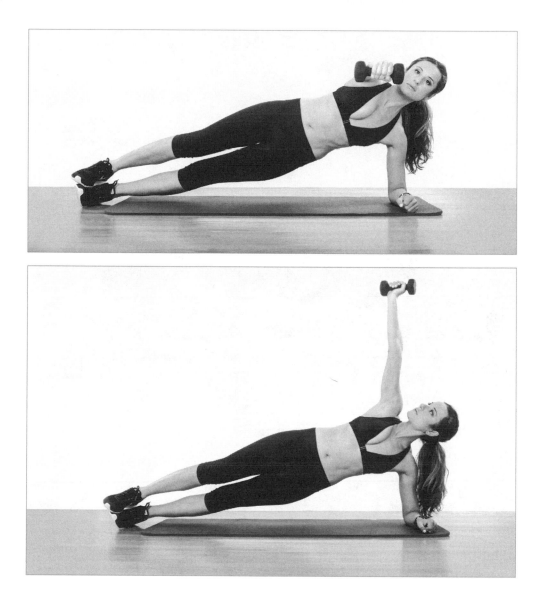

Side Plank with Forward Arm Extension

Lie on your right side and your right forearm with your shoulders, hips, knees, and feet in alignment and your feet stacked on top of each other. Keep your core tight. Hold a dumbbell in your left hand and extend your arm forward in front of your body, then up toward the ceiling (keep your arm straight the whole way). Return to the starting position. Repeat, then after working this side for a set, switch to the other.

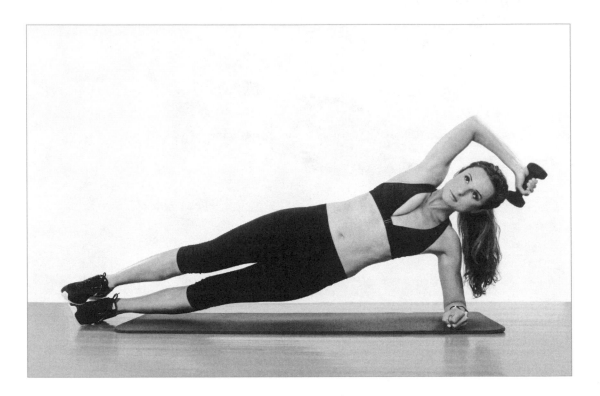

Side Plank with Triceps Extension

Start in a side plank position on your right side (see above), keeping your abs engaged and your body in a straight line. Hold a dumbbell in your left hand and extend your left arm up in the air above your shoulder, keeping your left elbow next to your left ear. From here, bend your elbow and bring the dumbbell down and back behind your head. Raise your arm back up and repeat. Once you have completed a set in a right side plank, switch to a left side plank.

Lateral Raise

Stand with your feet shoulder-width apart and hold a dumbbell in each hand with your arms hanging down at your sides. Keep your arms straight and raise your arms up and out to the side to shoulder level but not beyond. At the top, your palms should face the floor. Lower your arms back down and repeat.

THE CRANK-IT-UP CHALLENGE: Do single-arm lateral raises (one at a time) to work your core more.

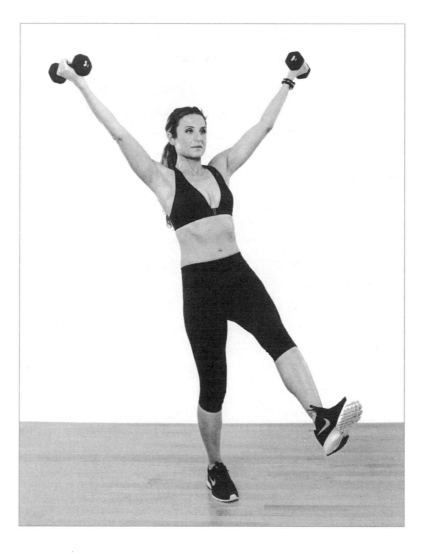

Standing W-press

Stand with your feet shoulder-width apart, holding a dumbbell in each hand. Bring your elbows to touch your sides, then raise your arms up into the letter W (so that the weights are above your shoulders but your elbows are still bent) then slowly bring them back down to your sides.

THE CRANK-IT-UP CHALLENGE: Try doing this while lifting one leg off the ground—a great way to challenge your balance and work your core at the same time. Don't forget to switch legs and work both sides. Also increase the weight of the dumbbell as you get stronger.

Extended-Arm Bicep Curl with Knee Raise

Stand with your feet shoulder-width apart and your arms extended out to shoulder height, with your palms facing up. While holding dumbbells, do arm curls by bending at the elbows and keeping your wrists locked. As you curl your arms in, raise your right knee up toward your chest to a 90-degree angle. As you release your curl back to a straight, extended arm, lower your knee back to the standing position. Continue doing curls with a right-knee raise until you are halfway through your set. Do your remaining curls by raising the left knee.

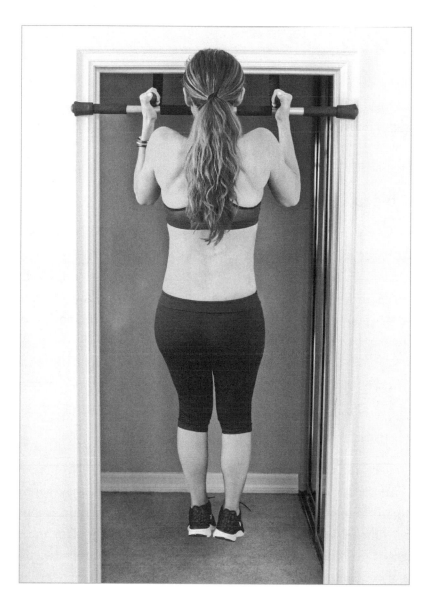

Close-Grip Pull-Up

Hang from your pull-up bar with your hands right next to each other on the bar; your palms should be facing you. Pull your body up until your chin is over the bar, keeping your elbows tucked in close toward your body. (*Note:* This is easier than the Wide-Grip Pull-Up. If you can't accomplish this, even just hanging and bringing yourself up an inch helps build strength.)

Bicep Curl

Stand with your feet hip-width apart and hold a dumbbell in each hand with your palms facing forward. Keeping your abs in and your knees slightly bent, bend your arms and bring your palms toward your shoulders in a bicep curl. Move your arms to the side to work your biceps at a different angle.

In-Out Bicep Curl

With this move, you first curl your arms in front of your body and then you curl them out to the side. Start by standing with your feet shoulder-width apart, holding a dumbbell in each hand down at your sides; your palms should be facing your body. Curl both weights up to your chest, bending your elbows and rotating your palms to face your chest. Lower your arms back to the starting position. Next curl your hands up on the outside of your body (at a diagonal angle) toward your shoulders. Keep your elbows close to your body. Lower your hands back to the starting position and repeat.

Bicep-Shoulder Combo

This is essentially an overhead shoulder press on one side above your head and a bicep curl on the other side. To do it, stand with your feet shoulder-width apart and hold a dumbbell in each hand. The right dumbbell should extend down at your side. Your left arm should be extended up from your shoulder and bent at the elbow at a 90-degree angle so that your dumbbell is next to your head. With your right hand, curl your dumbbell up and in toward your shoulder. At the same time, press your left dumbbell up over your head until your arm is fully extended. Continue to do bicep curls on your right side while doing an overhead shoulder press on your left. After completing your reps on that side, perform them on the other.

7

Cutting to the Core

Many people have the wrong idea about what it means to develop core strength: they think it's all about developing a six-pack or an eight-pack or washboard abs. There's no question that a well-defined midsection looks fabulous in a midriff top or a bikini. Yet it's about so much more than any of that. What would you do without core strength? Nothing very well, as Jen likes to say. If you really want to develop a strong core, you need to challenge all the muscles in the abdomen—the rectus abdominis (the two bands of muscle that run down the center of your abdomen), the transverse abdominis (the muscle that wraps horizontally around your lower abdomen), and the internal and the external obliques (which form the innermost and outermost layers of muscle that run down the sides of your waist). In other words, to build true core strength, you need to work the muscles that are deep inside your core, not just the superficial muscles.

Building a strong core is important for lots of reasons. For starters, the muscles in your core, along with the muscles in your back, provide the girdle or corset that supports your entire body. Developing a powerful core can reduce your risk of

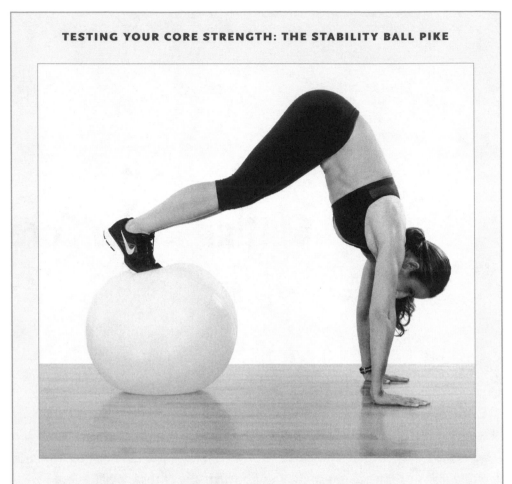

The stability ball pike is a true test of core strength because it requires so many muscles to work together. To do it, place your toes onto an exercise ball while extending your body out from the ball and assuming a push-up position with your palms on the floor. Slowly move the ball in a steady, controlled motion toward your hands, using the front portion of your feet. On the way in, get into the pike position by pushing your hips and butt up toward the ceiling. Keep your legs straight and contract your abs. From the pike position, move the ball back out and repeat. Practice doing a set of 15 pikes three times a week, and track your improvement in terms of how high you can do the pike or how many you can do with proper form and balance.

experiencing lower back pain or injury. By contrast, neglecting these crucial muscles can shortchange you of the stability your body needs for a variety of movements. After all, the muscles in your core help with balance, agility, and posture, yet some women have focused exclusively on doing crunches (which just work the superficial ab muscles) and shirked core-stabilization moves, compromising their overall core strength and lower-back stability in the process. This can throw their posture out of whack, weaken their athletic performance, and increase the risk of lower back strain and pain.

The core is also where your strength and power originates for playing sports, generating explosive movements, and performing other physical feats (like lifting or carrying items). Having a weak core is like turning off your body's power center and trying to rely only on satellite forms of energy instead—not a good idea! As a bonus, training your core muscles will make your body appear leaner and more streamlined overall.

Keep in mind, though, that if ripped abs are your goal, no amount of core training guarantees you'll get them. You will need to modify your diet, too, so that you're eating only clean and lean foods, especially if you're carrying extra pounds around your belly. Have you ever heard the expression "Abs are made in the kitchen, not the gym"? The truth is they're made in both places. But many people don't realize that sticking with lean proteins and lots of veggies will help them get to the prize of a hard core. (To help those newly defined muscles show through, you'll want to consume plenty of diuretic foods and teas to help you avoid or get rid of fluid retention.) Ramping up your cardio workouts will make a huge difference, too, because it will help you burn off the superficial layer of belly fat as well as fat elsewhere on your body.

If you take these steps and you do a variety of core-strengthening exercises regularly, you will probably begin to see a difference in the tone and definition of your midsection within three weeks. That's a pretty quick payoff on your investment.

Basic Plank

Lie facedown on the floor and raise yourself up onto your forearms and your toes, keeping the middle of your forearms right underneath your shoulders. Keep your hips raised and your back flat so your body resembles a plank that's parallel to the floor. Squeeze your abs and butt while doing this, and hold the position for 30 to 60 seconds, as long as you can.

Variations

Plank with One Arm Extension

Start in a basic push-up position, with your weight on your hands and the balls of your feet. Extend one arm straight out in front of your head. Hold this position for as long as you can, then bring your arm back to the floor. Switch arms.

Plank with Alternating Knee-to-Elbow Rotations

Start in a full push-up (or plank) position with your hands directly under your shoulders. Drive your right knee under and across your body to meet your left elbow, then return your right foot to the floor. Switch legs and repeat. Continue alternating back and forth. (*Note:* This is a great exercise for your oblique muscles!)

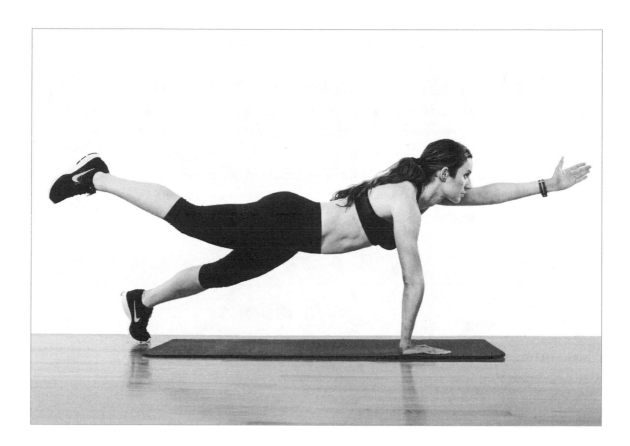

Plank with One Leg Extension

Start in a basic push-up position, then lift one foot a couple of inches off the ground into the air. Keep both legs completely straight and don't let your midsection sag! Hold this position for 30 to 60 seconds (or as long as you can), then return the first foot to the floor and switch legs.

THE CRANK-IT-UP CHALLENGE: Try the Bird Dog, in which you simultaneously lift your right leg straight up behind you and extend your left arm straight out in front of you, then switch sides.

Basic Crunch

Lie on your back on the floor, bend your knees, and place your feet flat on the floor hip-width apart. Place your hands behind your head with your elbows extended wide and parallel to the floor and keep your chin lifted. Press your lower back against the floor, then exhale and contract your abs by pulling your belly button toward your spine as you lift your shoulders off the floor, with your head (and gaze) facing the ceiling. When you get to the top, pause for a couple of seconds, then inhale as you slowly lower your shoulders to the floor. Repeat.

Variations

Bicycle Crunch

Lie on your back with your feet together and extend your legs straight out in front of you, a few inches off the floor. Lace your hands together behind your ears and open your elbows out wide to the sides. Keep your left leg straight and bend your right knee toward your upper body as you twist and touch your left elbow to your right knee. Then twist and turn so your right leg straightens and your left knee bends and touches your right elbow. Keep bringing your opposite elbow to the opposite knee in a slow, controlled fashion.

Reverse Crunch

Lie on your back with your knees bent, your feet flat on the floor, and your arms extended out to your sides at shoulder level, palms flat on the floor. Lift your feet off the floor and raise your knees directly above your hips (your knees should be together and bent at a 90-degree angle). Exhale and slowly raise your hips off the floor, rolling your spine up as you bring your knees toward your head. When you lift your spine as high as you can, pause briefly, then inhale and slowly lower your spine and hips back to the starting position (with your knees above your hips). Repeat.

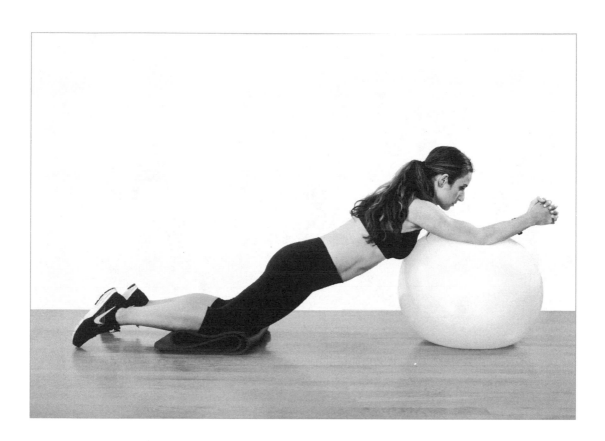

Stability Ball Roll-In

While your weight is on your toes or knees, place your forearms on a stability ball. From here, roll the ball forward slightly while keeping your abs engaged, then roll the ball back to the starting position. Repeat and continue at a steady pace.

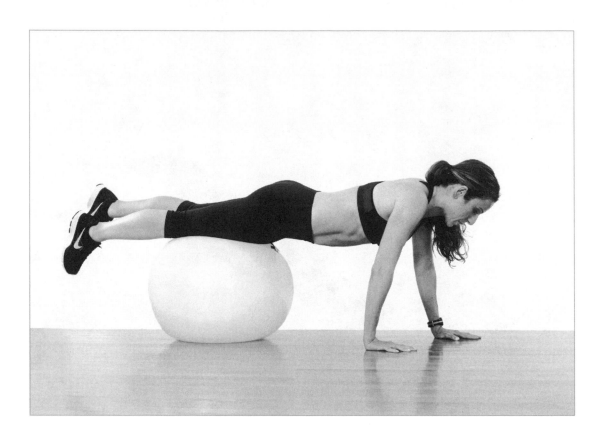

Body Roll-Out

Start with your chest on the stability ball and place your hands on the floor in front of the ball. Walk your hands and your body forward until your toes are the only part of your body on the ball. Then, use your hands to walk yourself back to the starting position. Repeat.

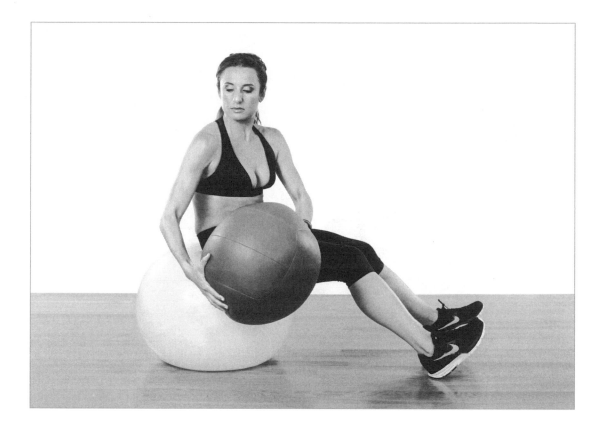

Side-to-Side Ball Crunch

Lie on your back with your knees bent and hold a medicine ball in your hands, extending it above your head toward the ceiling. Exhale as you sit up, contracting your abs and bringing the ball forward and down toward the floor; then, rotate your torso and the ball to the right. Bring your torso back to the center, then lie back on the floor. Next time, sit up and rotate your torso and the ball to the left side, return to center, then lie back on the floor. Repeat the pattern.

THE CRANK-IT-UP CHALLENGE: Perform this on a stability ball.

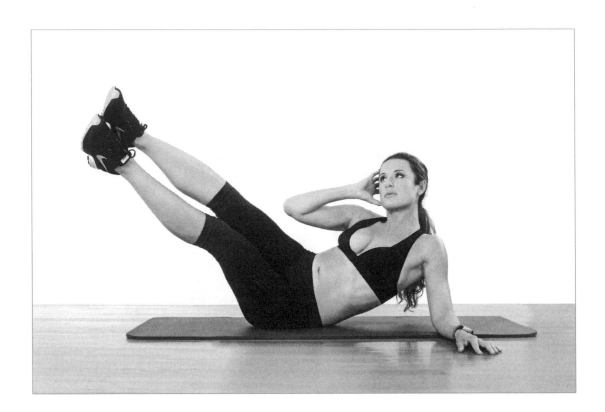

Side V-up

Lie on your right side with your legs stacked and bent at a 30-degree angle from your hips. Place your right hand behind your head and your left arm on the floor. From this position, engage your core and lift your torso and your extended legs off the floor, bringing your torso toward your legs. Release yourself from this position without letting your torso or legs fully touch the ground, then repeat on the other side.

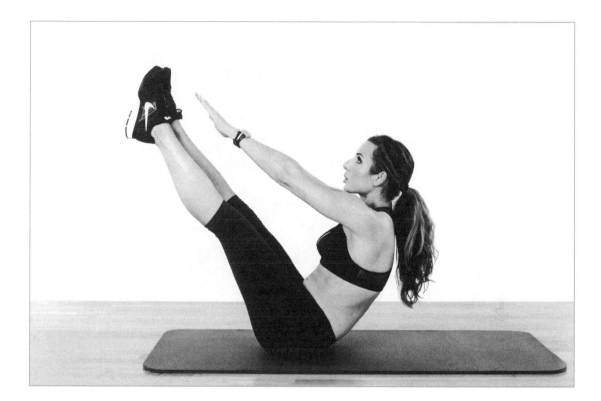

V-up

Lie on your back with your legs together and extended, and arms long and out to your sides at 90-degree angles. While keeping your back flat, use your abs to sit up while drawing your knees in toward your chest. As you sit up, wrap your arms around your knees. Hold for a count of one, then release your body from this position, extending your legs out straight and lowering your torso toward the floor—but without lowering either your legs or your torso completely to the ground. From this position, repeat.

THE CRANK-IT-UP CHALLENGE: Do this move while keeping your legs entirely straight and reach your fingers toward your toes.

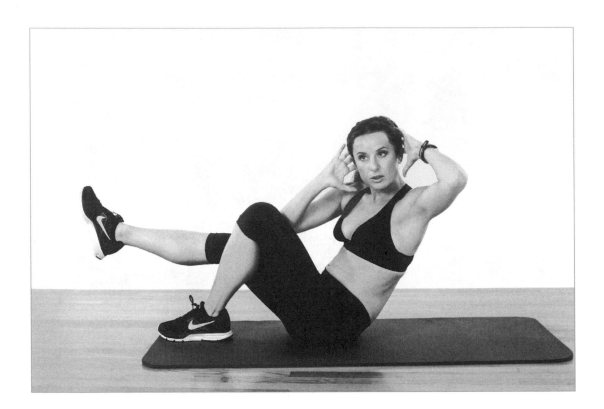

Vertical Sit-Up with Crossover Elbow to Knee

Lie on your back with your left leg bent and your right leg extended and raised a few inches in the air; your fingertips should be behind your head. From this position, tighten your abs and bend from the waist to bring your upper body off the ground and toward your bent knee; return to the floor. Continue to work this side of your body before switching to the other side (in which case you'll bend your left knee and straighten your right leg along the floor).

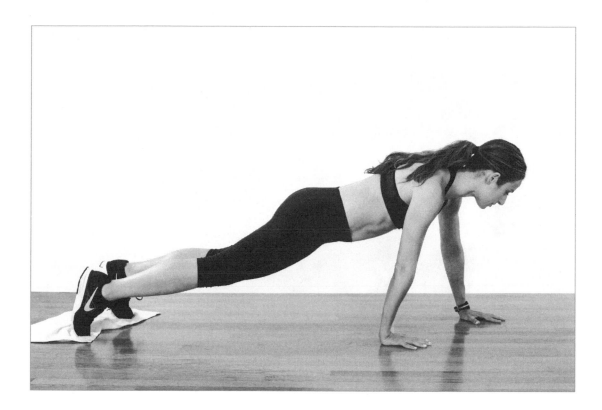

Plank Drag with Towel

Get into a plank or a push-up position and place a towel under both sets of toes. Your hands should be on the floor, directly under your shoulders, your back should be flat, and your abs engaged. Now drag your body across the room using your arms to pull your body weight and your toes to drag the towel (this forces stabilization of your core). Go to one end of the room and back, turning around when you reach each endpoint. (*Bonus:* Your floor will get dusted at the same time!)

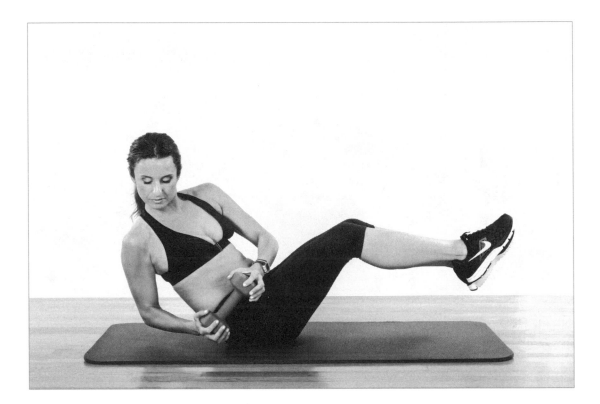

Russian Twist

Sit with your knees bent and your feet a few inches off the ground. Your torso should be leaning back at a 45-degree angle to the floor. Hold one dumbbell with both hands by using each hand to grasp each end. From this position, rotate as far as you can to the right side and touch the dumbbell to the ground, then rotate to the left side of your body and touch down. Repeat back and forth.

VARIATION: If you are just beginning and need more stability, you can keep your feet on the floor while rotating your torso.

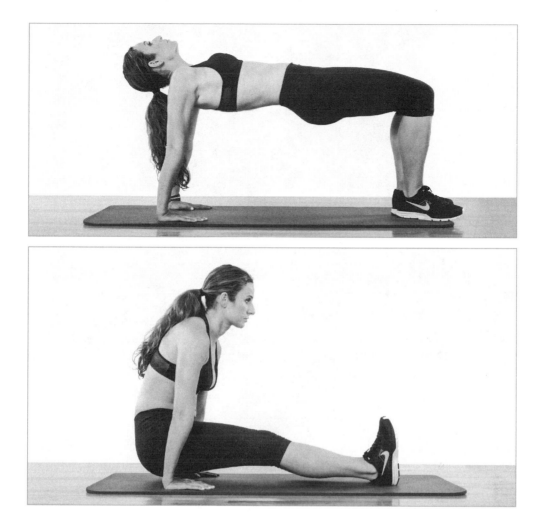

Reverse Tabletop

Get into a reverse tabletop position with your butt facing the floor and your torso parallel to the ceiling, your palms on the floor right underneath your shoulders, and your feet flat on the floor. Keep your fingers spread, your chin lifted off your chest, and your hips lifted toward the ceiling. Let your hips drop and bend from the waist at a 90-degree angle as you rock your butt down and back through your arms so that your butt ends up behind you and your legs are fully extended (you'll be resting on your heels). Pause in this position, then use your abs to thrust your hips forward through your arms and back up toward the ceiling to the original tabletop position. Repeat.

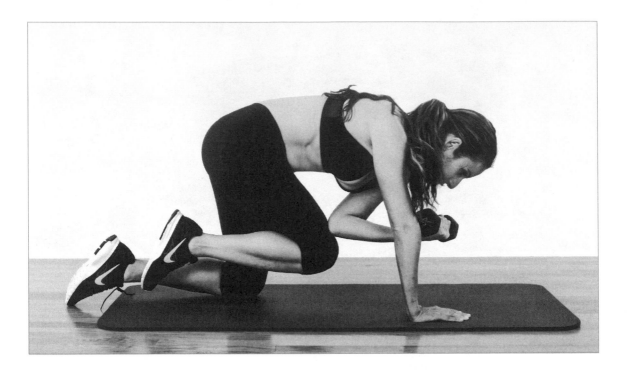

Tabletop with Elbow-to-Knee Crunch

Get into a traditional tabletop position with your hands and knees on the floor (your torso facing the floor and your butt facing the ceiling). Place your hands directly beneath your shoulders, and keep your back flat. Hold a light dumbbell in your right hand. From this position, extend your right arm out in front of you. At the same time extend your left leg straight out behind you. Next crunch your abs, bringing your right elbow in to meet your left knee in the middle of your body (near your belly button). Extend them both again and repeat. Work one side before switching to the other side. Remember to switch your dumbbell to the other hand!

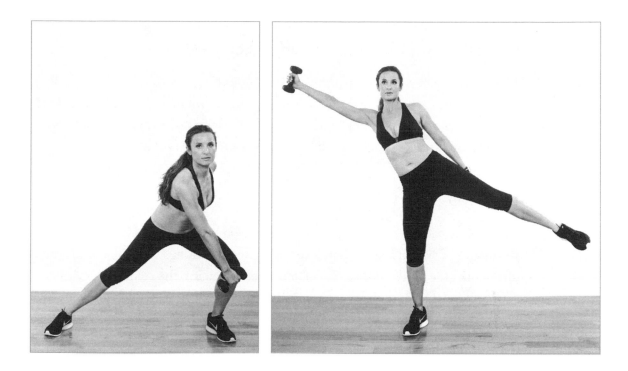

Lateral Lunge with Half X

Stand with your feet hip-width apart and your toes turned slightly toward the corners of the room. Place a dumbbell in your left hand and step out with your right leg into a lateral (sideways) lunge, bending your knee as close to a 90-degree angle as possible. Next push out of your lunge into a half X by kicking your right leg out into a 45-degree angle from your standing leg while extending your left arm to the ceiling. Return to the starting position. Repeat. Change sides once you've completed a set.

Opposite Arm to Leg (a.k.a. Single-Leg Jackknife)

Lie on your back with your arms extended straight behind your head on the floor. Lift your torso, your left leg, and your right arm simultaneously, and try to touch your left toes with your right hand. Return to the starting position (so you're lying down again) and repeat. Switch sides after you complete the set.

Leg Drop

Lie on your back with your legs together and your arms either at your sides with your palms down or under your lower back. Keep your legs straight and lift them to a 90-degree angle so the soles of your feet are facing the ceiling. Slowly lower your legs to the ground, keeping your knees slightly bent and letting your legs hover an inch or so off the ground for a count of one, then raise them back so they're perpendicular to the floor again. As you repeat this move, keep your abs tight and pulled back so that your spine is flush against the floor.

TIRE FLIPS

With this challenge, lower-body strength is crucial. If you've never done a tire flip, as in, flipping a large tire over—hey, you've got plenty of company there—be sure to start with a smaller, light tire or even a weight plate. Stand with your feet hip-width apart and your knees bent. Hinge forward from your hips and grasp the tire with both hands in an underhand position (palms against the tire's surface). Lift the tire, using your core and lower body for strength and keeping your abs tight (so you don't strain your back), then flip it over. Repeat. Gradually increase the size and weight of the tire, using the same good form.

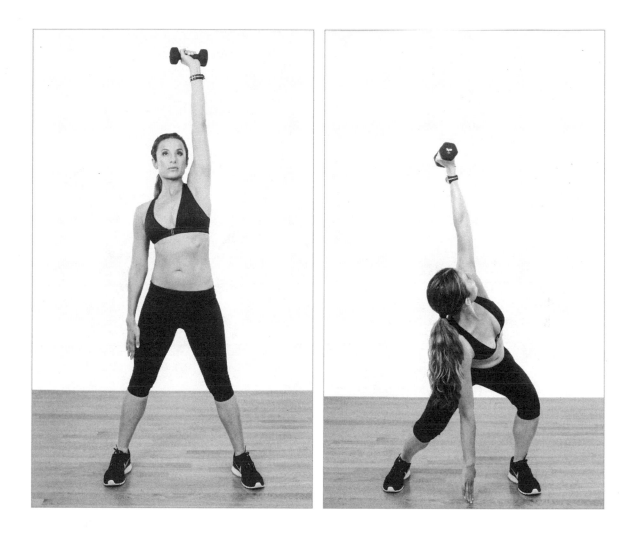

Windmill

Stand with your feet hip-width apart and hold a dumbbell in your right hand; extend it up toward the ceiling, keeping your right arm as straight as possible and your right elbow close to your right ear. Keeping your hips forward, rotate from your waist and reach the fingertips of your left hand down toward the floor, then stand back up to the starting position. Repeat. Once you've done a complete set, switch sides.

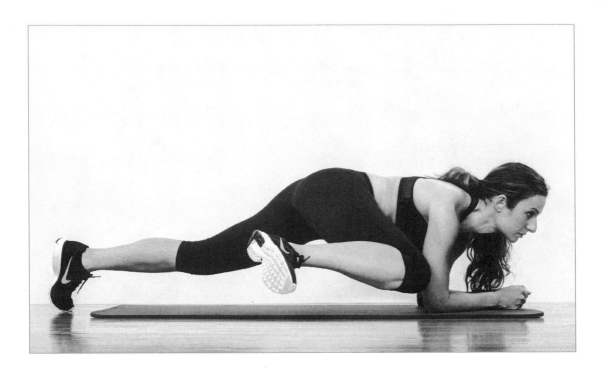

Spider-Man Plank Crunch

Get into a modified plank position with your forearms on the ground and your elbows directly under your shoulders. Your core should be engaged, and your body should stay in a straight line. Drive your right knee up toward your right elbow (your knee should track along the outside of your body); you should feel your hip opening up as you pull your knee toward your elbow. Return to the plank position, and repeat with the left side. Continue alternating sides.

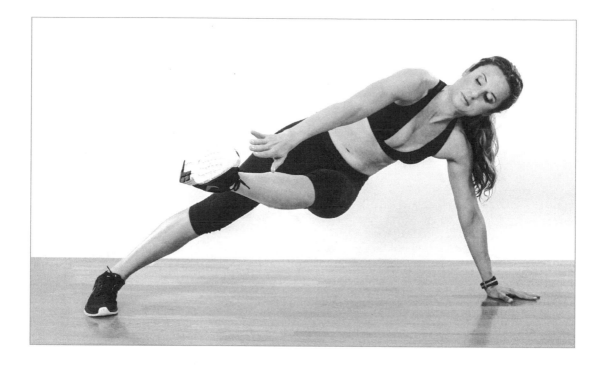

Cross Toe Touch

Get into a plank position with your hands on the floor directly under your shoulders and your core engaged. Cross your right leg under your body, and lift your left hand to touch your right toes as the right foot comes under and through, then return the left hand and the right foot to the starting position. Next cross your left foot under your body and touch it with your right hand. Continue to alternate legs and hands. (*Warning:* This is a hard one!)

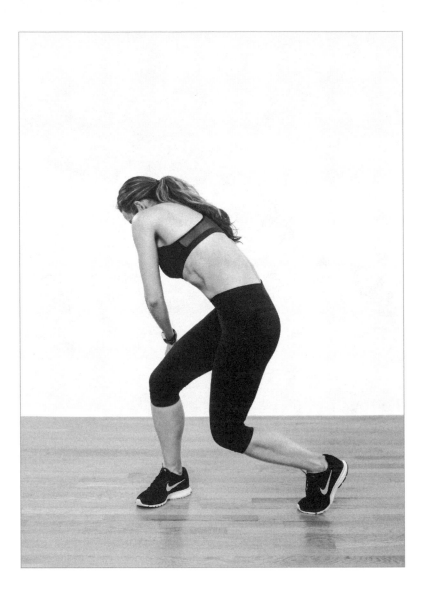

Woodchopper

Stand with your feet hip-width apart and your body weight on your left leg. Start by holding a dumbbell in both hands (one hand grasping each end) up by your left shoulder. Next, rotate your body and your arms to make a chopping motion with the dumbbell down toward your right hip. Allow your feet and knees to pivot with the rotation. Raise the dumbbell back up to your left shoulder and repeat. Switch sides after you've completed a full set.

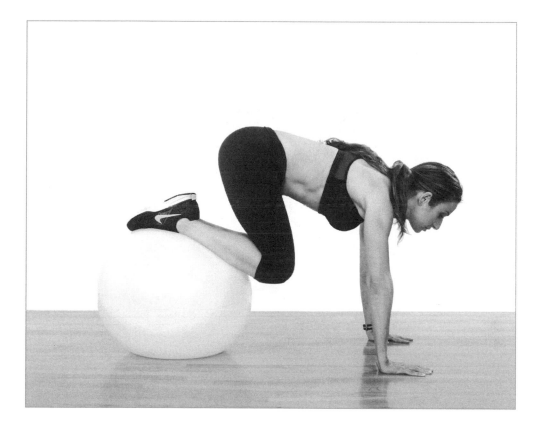

Leg Pull-In with a Ball

Get into a push-up position with the tops of your feet resting on a stability ball and your hands on the ground. From here, pull your knees in to your chest, rolling the ball toward your chest as you go. Roll the ball back out by extending your legs. Engage your core, and keep your neck straight with your eyes focused on the ground. Repeat.

THE QUICKIE CORE WORKOUT

If you want to concentrate on developing and strengthening your core—or if you want to gain the power you'll need to do a Stability Ball Pike (the ultimate core challenge, see page 122)—do this intense core workout three times a week. You will do 4 rounds of the following five exercises in this pattern:

1st round: Do each exercise for 60 seconds.

2nd round: Do each exercise for 50 seconds.

3rd round: Do each exercise for 40 seconds.

4th round: Do each exercise for 30 seconds.

(Use your smartphone, a stopwatch, or an egg timer if you don't have a partner to do the timing for you.)

1. Body Roll-Out

2. Side-to-Side Ball Crunch

3. V-up

4. Russian Twist

5. Leg Drop

THE 300 ABS

Remember Gerard Butler, who led a few hundred Spartans into battle in the epic movie *300*? If you want abs like his, try this workout, which happens to have 300 reps total.

30 Basic Crunches

20 Bicycle Crunches

15 Opposite Arm to Leg (right side)

15 Opposite Arm to Leg (left side)

20 Reverse Crunches

15 Plank with Alternating Knee-to-Elbow Rotations

30 Crunches

15 Plank with Alternating Knee-to-Elbow Rotations

40 Russian Twists

30 Bicycle Crunches

15 Side V-ups (right side)

20 Reverse Crunches

15 Side V-ups (left side)

20 Leg Drops

8
Getting a Leg Up on Strength

Who among us doesn't want firm, shapely, powerful thighs and calves, not to mention a strong, toned derriere? Having robust, capable legs can help us walk, run, jump, bend, cycle, climb, and move through other activities of daily life much more comfortably, steadily, and agilely. One way or another, we rely on our legs for almost everything we do. No wonder having great gams is practically a universal item on women's wish lists for their bodies! The good news is they are attainable! In fact, with the right moves and the right reps, you'll see faster results in building leg strength than almost any other part of your body. Plus, you can get rid of the body bits that may have bothered you for years and develop legs that can (literally!) kick ass.

Not only will your legs look better when you consistently treat them to the right workout, but you'll also be doing your whole body a favor by building strength from the waist down. After all, your legs are your basic transportation system—they give you the means and the power to get around—so you'll want to develop greater strength and stamina for walking, running, stepping, and climbing. Most of your

One of the easiest ways to improve lower-body (muscle and bone) strength is to climb several flights of stairs each day. The energy required for climbing steps comes almost exclusively from the legs. To improve the effects of stair-climbing, try taking the stairs two at a time. This forces the body to perform a lunging movement, which can increase strength in your thighs in particular.

daily actions involve your legs, and your leg muscles are among the most important muscles in your body for balance, stability, and overall power. So you'll want to develop strong legs to stand on, physically and mentally (the two often go together). It's also important to strengthen your buttocks (a.k.a. your glutes) to help you have a steady, strong gait when you walk. Plus, the better conditioned your legs are now, the greater mobility you'll have as you get older, and you'll have a lower risk of developing injuries in your knees, hips, and ankles. All in all, doing well-rounded leg workouts regularly builds lean muscle mass, supports bone density (decreasing your risk of osteoporosis), reduces stress on your bones and joints, and improves balance, making you less susceptible to falling (a big plus as you age).

Yet, many people have imbalances between key muscle groups in their legs—namely, between the quadriceps (the muscles that run down the front of each thigh) and the hamstrings (the muscles that extend from the base of your butt to the backs of your knees). Some people's quads are stronger than their hamstrings, while others have the opposite scenario. Similarly, some people have tighter hip flexors and more flexible glutes. The problem is, if you're constantly relying on one set of muscles to pick up the slack for another—which can become an ingrained habit—you can burn out the ones that are doing most of the work; this then causes trickle-down stress for adjacent muscles, which can lead to injuries in those muscles. Or you can develop muscle strains or tendonitis in the overworked muscles themselves.

That's why it's important to include exercises that challenge opposing muscle groups in your leg workouts and moves that work both sides of the body to prevent and correct muscle imbalances. (Maintaining proper form is also crucial for preventing or readjusting muscle inequities.) The best leg workouts train the quads,

> ### BOX JUMPS
>
> To build the lower-body power and strength you'll need to do box jumps, start by doing lots of jump squats . . . and more jump squats. As you get stronger, try exploding higher and higher off the ground, making sure to land softly each time. Once you're ready for the next challenge, try jumping up onto a step and back down to the ground using the same technique (swing your arms upward to gain momentum). Once you've mastered the step, try a higher platform or box, making sure to maintain control on the explosive upward move as well as the landing. Continue progressing in height as long as you can. You can also increase your reps to build extra strength.

the hamstrings, the adductors (the muscles on your inner thighs), the abductors (the muscles on your outer thighs), the calf muscles, the hip flexors (the muscles on your upper thighs, just below your hip bones, that allow you to lift your knees and bend at the waist), and the gluteus maximus and gluteus minimus (a.k.a. the glutes). The hip flexors are often overworked since we use them in everyday activities like standing up and sitting down, so it's important to stretch these often-tight muscles properly.

The exercises that follow will give you the legwork you need to get strong, healthy gams. Make them a regular part of your life and you'll feel and see the results you crave before you know it.

Front Lunge with Dumbbell Pass-Through

Stand with your feet shoulder-width apart and your toes facing forward. Hold a dumbbell in your left hand and step forward with your right foot into a lunge; your front (right) leg should be bent at a 90-degree angle and your back (left) heel should be lifted. While you are in the lunge, pass the dumbbell under your front leg to your right hand. Push yourself back into the standing position. Next do a lunge on your left leg, passing the dumbbell under your left leg from your right hand to your left hand. Return to the standing position and repeat.

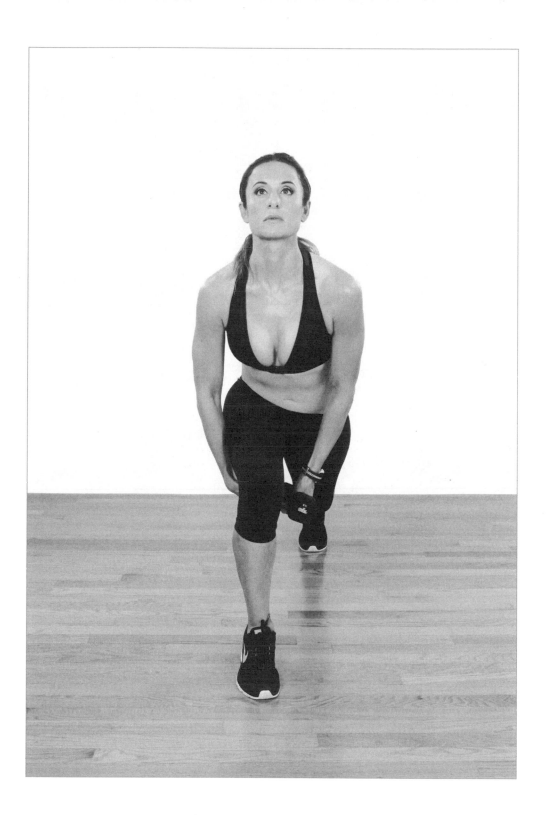

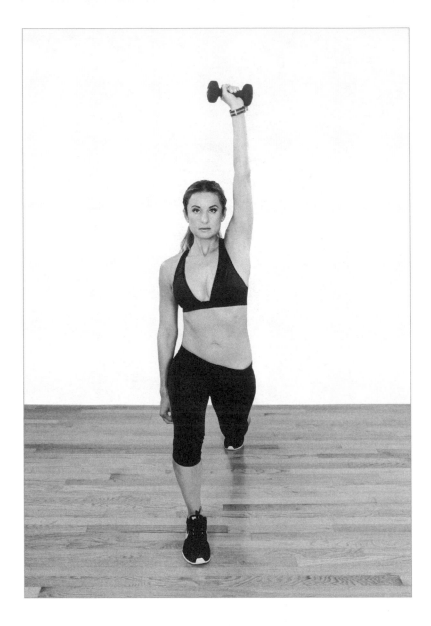

Front Lunge with Single-Dumbbell Overhead Press

Take a dumbbell in your right hand and extend it up and over your head toward the ceiling. Lunge forward with your left leg while your right arm is still extended; keep your chest lifted as you do this. Return to the standing position, lower the weight, and repeat. Switch sides after you have finished a complete set on this first side.

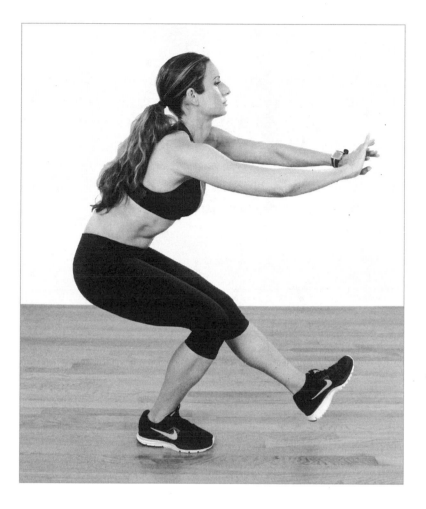

Single-Leg Squat

Stand on your right leg with a bench or chair behind you (to use as a safety net) and lift your left foot a couple of inches off the ground. Keep your weight on the heel of your standing foot; be careful not to lean forward or let your right knee move past your toes. Slowly lower yourself down into a squat until your glutes barely tap the seat, exhale, and stand straight up on the right leg. Continue for a full set on the right leg, and then switch over to the left. (*Note:* If you need extra help in the balance department or if you're just beginning, lightly hold onto the back of a chair or actually sit on the seat as you squat for extra support.)

THE CRANK-IT-UP CHALLENGE: Once you can do this move easily, try to lower yourself until your knees are bent at 90-degree angles before returning to standing.

Sumo Squat Jump

Stand with your feet slightly more than hip-width apart and your feet pointed out toward the corners of the room. Place your hands on your hips or straight out in front of you; keep your shoulders back and your chest lifted. Lower your body down into a deep squat, then drive yourself up into a jump, pushing from the balls of your feet; your legs should straighten out as your feet leave the floor. As you land back on your feet, lower yourself back down into another sumo squat and repeat.

VARIATION: Do the same move without the jump (a great option for those with knee injuries).

Side Step to Side Kick

Stand with an elevated platform (at least 12 inches high) on your right side and hold a dumbbell in each hand. Step with your right foot onto the platform and kick your left leg out to the side as you do so. Return to the standing position on the floor, and repeat for a complete set on the right side. Then switch to the left.

THE CRANK-IT-UP CHALLENGE: Add a bicep curl on both sides before you step down from the platform.

Offset Split Lunge with Shoulder Press

Stand with your feet shoulder-width apart and rest your right foot behind you on a step or platform. Hold a dumbbell in your right hand up in front of your right shoulder, with your knuckles facing your shoulder. While your right foot is on the platform, bend your left knee at a 90-degree angle into a lunge, then push up from the lunge until your left leg is fully extended. As you push up, press the dumbbell up above your head into a shoulder press. Lower the dumbbell as you return to the lunge. (Throughout the sequence, remember to keep your chest up, your shoulders back, and your knees in line with your toes.) Repeat an entire set on this side. Once you are done working your left leg, switch to lunges on the right side.

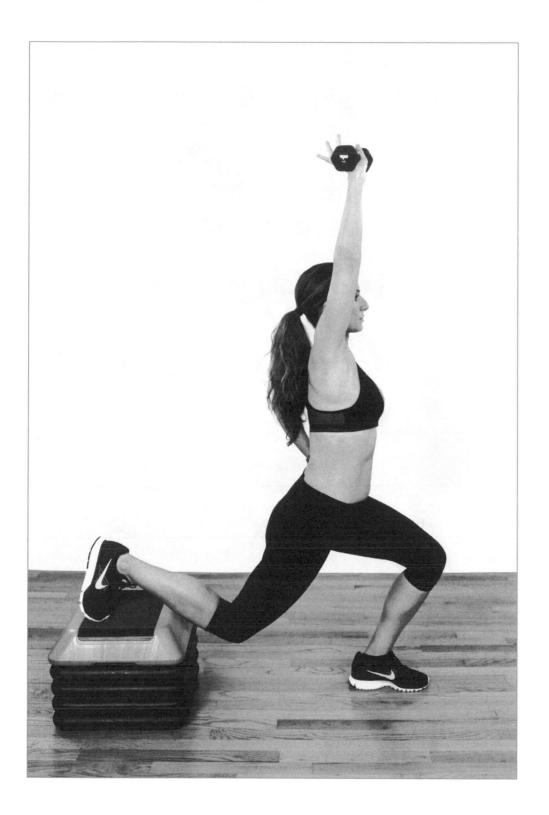

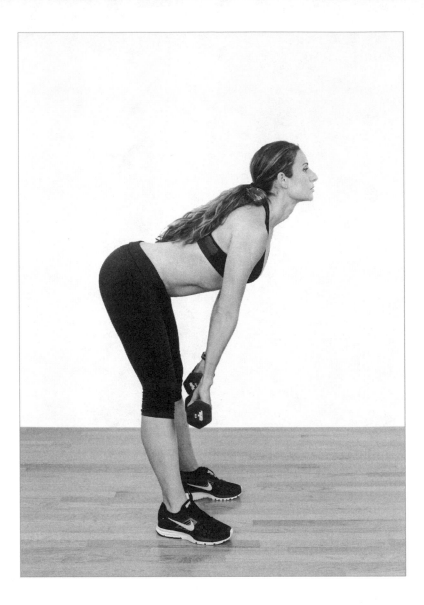

Deadlift

Stand with your feet hip-width apart and hold two dumbbells straight down in front of you. Hinge forward from your hips until the weights are just below your knees. Make sure to keep your back flat, your chest lifted, and your knees slightly bent. Once you are in this bent-over position, return to the standing position, keeping your core engaged and squeezing your butt as you lift up to standing. Repeat.

Deadlift with Rotation Twist

Stand with your feet shoulder-width apart, and hold a dumbbell in each hand in front of your thighs. Hinge forward from the hips, keeping your back flat as you lower the dumbbells toward the floor. As you squeeze your glutes, bend your elbows and lift your arms to a goalpost position (your elbows at shoulder level, with your knuckles pointed toward the ceiling) as you come to a full standing position. While keeping your arms in the goalpost position, rotate your torso slightly to the right, then return to center. Repeat the entire move on the left side. Continue alternating sides throughout the set.

Single-Leg Deadlift

Stand with your feet hip-width apart and a dumbbell in each hand; the dumbbells should be extended straight in front of your thighs. Extend your right leg behind you so that it is raised about a foot off the ground. From here, hinge forward from your hips, keeping your back flat, and lower your weights until they are below your knees. As you do this, your extended leg should rise so that it stays in line with your body. From here, return to an upright position, squeezing your butt as you do. Your extended leg will lower back down, but it should not touch the ground. Do a full set with the right leg raised before switching to your other leg.

Squat with Overhead Press

Stand with your feet hip-width apart, holding a dumbbell in each hand up by your shoulders. Your palms should be facing out in front of you. While engaging your core, lower yourself into a squat so your legs bend to a 90-degree angle. As you push up out of the squat, press the dumbbells up above your head until your arms are fully extended. From here, lower the weights back down to your shoulders as you lower yourself into another squat. Repeat the sequence.

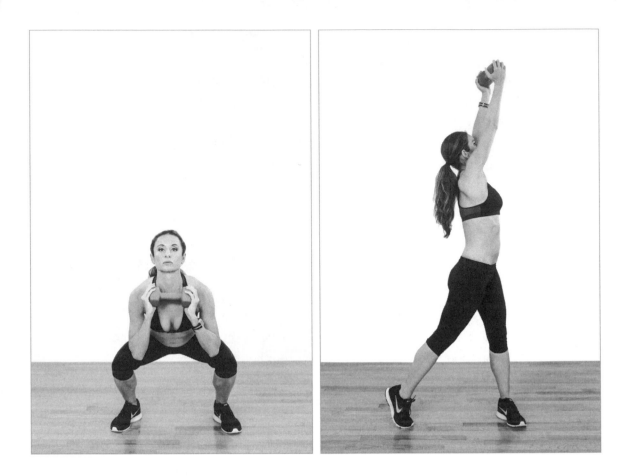

Deep Squat with Overhead Rotation

Stand with your feet hip-width apart and hold a heavy dumbbell (place your hands at each end of the weight) at chest level in front of you. While engaging your core, lower your body into a squat, bending your knees past a 90-degree angle and keeping your body weight on your heels and your torso leaning slightly forward. As you push yourself back up to a standing position, turn your body to the right by lifting and pivoting your left heel, and fully extend your arms overhead toward the back of the room (your core should be engaged). Bring your body back to the center as you lower yourself down into another squat and move the dumbbell back to the starting position. Go back into your squat and repeat on the left side. Continue alternating sides.

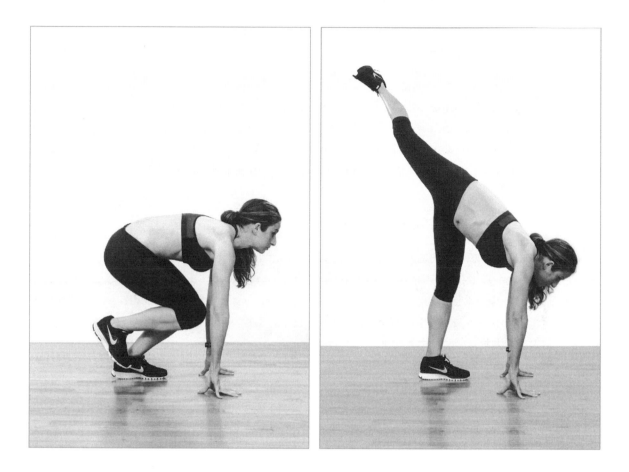

Reverse Leg Press

Starting with your feet shoulder-width apart, bend your knees slightly and lean into a forward fold position so that your chest is toward your thighs and your hands are on the floor. From here, extend your right heel up behind you toward the ceiling, keeping your right leg straight. Remember to keep your belly button pulled in and your left foot firmly pressed into the floor with your body weight in the middle of your foot. Bring your right leg back down and tap the floor before sending it behind you toward the ceiling again. Return to the starting position. Continue to squat and press your heel toward the ceiling on one side for a full set, then switch to the other leg.

Offset Squat

Stand with your feet hip-width apart and your arms extended down at your sides. Hold a dumbbell in your right hand. Engage your core and lower your body into a squat, bending your knees at a 90-degree angle with your body weight on your heels and your torso leaning slightly forward. Do a set of squats with the dumbbell on your right side, and then switch to the left and do a set.

Lateral Walk-Out with Band

Stand on a straight resistance band that has handles with your feet hip-width apart, holding the ends of the band at your sides to provide resistance. Step out to the left with your left foot, and then bring it back in to a hip-width stance. Repeat with your right foot. Continue to alternate feet.

Step-Up

Find a step, bench, or chair that will allow your knee to bend as close to a 90-degree angle as possible when you place your foot on it in front of you. To start, hold a dumbbell in each hand, and step up onto the step, bench, or chair with the right foot, then the left; bring both feet completely onto the elevated surface. Return to the starting position by leading with the right foot, stepping down to the floor, then step down with the left, until you have both feet on the ground. Repeat until you have done a full set by alternating stepping up with the right foot then the left.

VARIATION (ONE-LEGGED STEP-UP): Stand with your feet shoulder-width apart facing a step, bench, or chair. Hold a dumbbell in your right hand at your side; keep your left hand free. From here, step up onto the platform with your right leg, driving your left knee up toward your chest as you do so. Keep your right foot on the step, and lower your left foot to tap the floor behind you, then drive the left knee up again. Continue to tap and raise your left leg at a steady pace for a full set. Once you are done stepping on the right side, switch to the left. Remember to switch your dumbbell to the left side, as well.

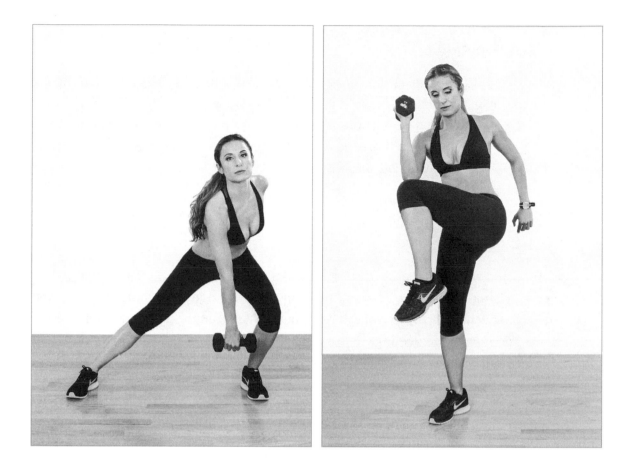

Lateral Lunge with Knee-to-Elbow Rotation

Stand with your feet hip-width apart and your toes pointing out toward the corners of the room. Hold a dumbbell in your left hand and step out with your right foot into a lateral (sideways) lunge, bending your knee as close to a 90-degree angle as possible, with your left hand reaching down toward your right foot. As you push yourself out of the lunge, drive your right knee to meet your left elbow in the middle of your body. Make sure to engage your abs throughout this entire motion. Uncurl and release back to the standing position, and continue doing right-side lunges. Once you have finished, switch to the left side.

Alternating Lunge

Stand with your feet shoulder-width apart and your toes facing forward; hold a dumbbell in each hand at your sides. Step forward with your right foot into a lunge (get down low but don't let your knee extend past your toes); at this point, both legs should be bent at 90-degree angles with your back heel off the ground. Push back to the standing position. Step into the lunge with the left foot and repeat. Continue alternating legs.

Bulgarian Lunge

Stand with your feet shoulder-width apart, and rest your right foot behind you on a platform (or step) so that you are in an elevated lunge position. Hold a dumbbell in each hand up by your chest. With your right foot on the platform, bend your left knee to a 90-degree angle into a lunge. Push up from the lunge until your left leg is fully extended, then return to standing. Repeat. Once you have done a set with your left leg, switch to the right side.

Reverse Lunge with Kick

Hold a dumbbell in each hand and stand with your feet shoulder-width apart. Step back with your right foot into a lunge until both legs are bent at 90-degree angles; keep your shoulders back and your chest lifted. From here, push back up into a standing position while kicking your back leg forward into a waist-high kick. After the kick, lower yourself back into another reverse lunge. Do a complete set with one leg lunging before switching to the other.

THE CRANK-IT-UP CHALLENGE: Stand on a platform or step and do the lunge in reverse behind you so you're activating more muscle groups.

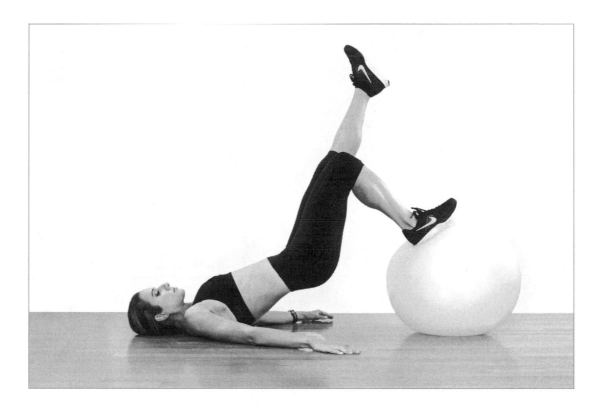

Hamstring Pull-In with Ball

Lie flat on your back with your ankles resting on top of a stability ball. Your arms should be extended straight out at your sides with your palms flat on the floor, and your legs extended straight. Lift your body up into a bridge until your butt is raised about a foot off the floor. Your body should form a straight line. Pull your knees in toward your chest, rolling the ball toward your butt as you go. Roll the ball back out to the starting position by straightening your legs. Repeat. Remember to keep your chest open and your arms on the ground throughout the move.

THE CRANK-IT-UP CHALLENGE: Do the same move but by pulling the ball in with one leg while the other leg is extended to the ceiling.

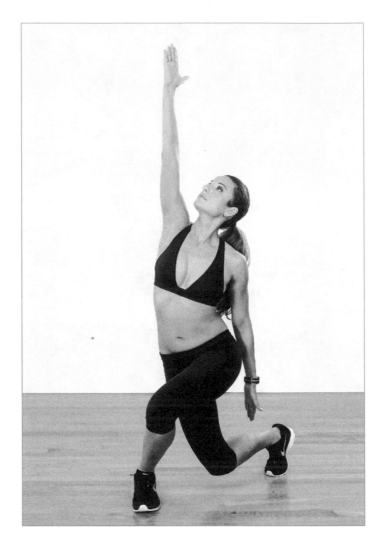

Curtsy Lunge

Stand with your feet shoulder-width apart and your toes facing forward. Hold a dumbbell in each hand—or if this is too much for you, perform the exercise without them. With your right foot, step back diagonally behind your left foot, bending both knees as close to a 90-degree angle as possible as you sit into the lunge. Return to the standing position. Repeat on the other side.

THE CRANK-IT-UP CHALLENGE: Use an elevated platform to increase the intensity. Start with both feet on the platform, then step back diagonally to the floor, in the same pattern as described above.

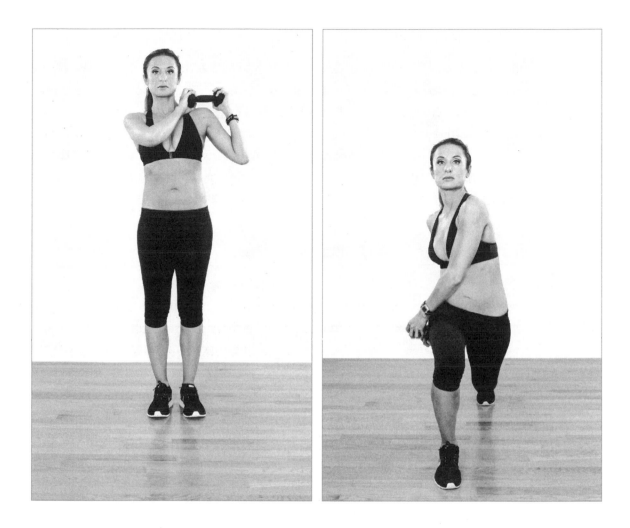

Forward Lunge with Woodchopper

Stand with your feet shoulder-width apart and use both hands to hold one dumbbell or medicine ball at your left shoulder. Step out into a forward lunge with your right leg, bending your right knee to a 90-degree angle. As you lunge, rotate the dumbbell down and over toward your right hip, making a chopping motion. As you push out of the lunge and back into a standing position, bring the dumbbell back up to your left shoulder. Do a set of these on your right side. Next do a set on your left side (with the dumbbell starting on your right shoulder).

Lateral Step-Out Squat

Stand with your feet shoulder-width apart and hold two dumbbells up next to your shoulders with your palms facing each other. (Alternatively, you can use a body bar resting across the back of your shoulders.) Step out into a squat to the right side with your right leg. Your knees should be bent as close to a 90-degree angle as possible and your knees should be in line with your toes (but behind them). Push yourself back up into a standing position. Repeat by stepping out on the left side. Continue doing lateral squats, alternating sides as you go.

Lateral Lunge with Dumbbell

Stand with your feet hip-width apart and your toes facing forward. Hold one heavier dumbbell (10 to 15 pounds) in front of your chest with both hands (by grasping each end of the dumbbell). Step to the right side into a lateral lunge, bending your knee as close to a 90-degree angle as you can. Keep your chest lifted and your right knee in line with your right toes (but behind them). Push yourself back into a standing position and repeat. Once you have done a set on your right side, switch to the left.

THE CRANK-IT-UP CHALLENGE: As you push out of the lunge, try lifting your foot a few inches off the ground and holding it for a count or two while standing on the other leg. You can also use a heavier weight.

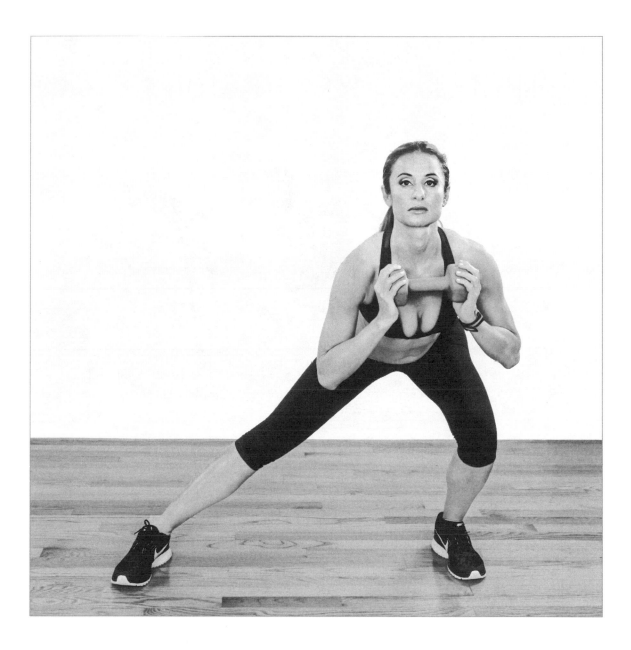

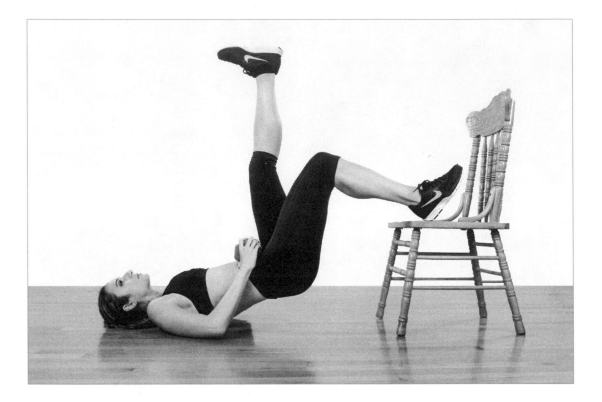

One-Legged Glute Bridge

Put a chair in front of your feet. Then, lie on your back on the floor, holding a single dumbbell (with your hands on each end) against your stomach. Bend your knees at 90-degree angles and rest your heels on the edge of the chair. Lift your left foot off the chair and up toward the ceiling, then drive your hips off the floor; your torso and left leg should form a straight line. Lower your hips back down to barely graze the ground, and repeat. Work one side before switching to your other leg. Remember to keep your abs tight and engaged throughout the exercise.

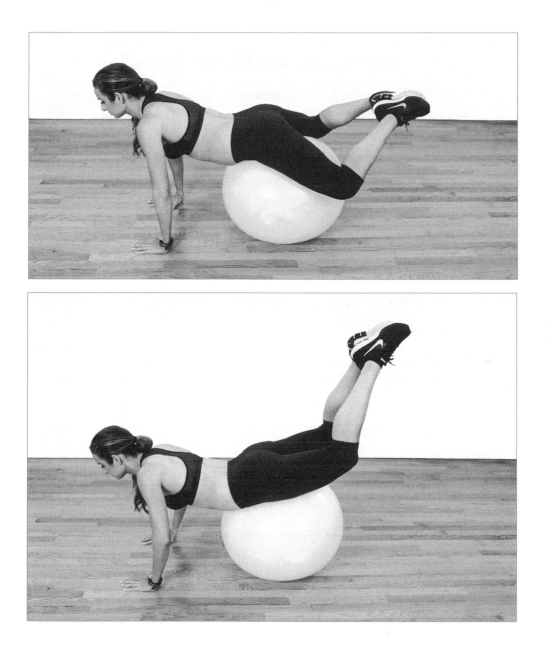

Frog Legs

Lie on a stability ball with your chest on the ball and your hands on the ground. From here, lift your legs off the ground, bend your knees, and bring your heels together behind you so they are touching (like a frog's). Lift and lower your legs while in this position with small, controlled motions.

THE QUICKIE LOWER-BODY WORKOUT

If you want to concentrate on strengthening and toning your lower body (especially the thighs and glutes), or if you want to gain a better sense of balance, do this intense but quick lower-body workout three times a week. As a bonus, the one-legged exercises will help even out muscle imbalances; we all have them to some extent. You will do 4 rounds of the following five exercises in this pattern:

1st round: Each exercise for 60 seconds.

2nd round: Each exercise for 50 seconds.

3rd round: Each exercise for 40 seconds.

4th round: Each exercise for 30 seconds.

1. One Legged Step-Up
2. Bulgarian Lunge
3. One-Legged Glute Bridge
4. Frog Legs
5. Reverse Leg Press

9

Assembling Strength

Now that you know what your current state of fitness is and where there's room for improvement, it's time to get to work! The good news is we've taken the guesswork out by providing you with a fitness power grid—the 4-3-2-1 Power Grid. Just as your local utility company has a power grid that distributes electrical power throughout your geographic region, your body has its own systems for generating and delivering power and energy. The difference is that your body relies on the mitochondria (the energy factories in your cells) for basic energy needs and muscle power when it comes to physical movement and strength. To develop your own high-voltage strength from head to toe, you'll want to follow our exercise power grid, which offers circuit workouts in a modified reverse pyramid format. Say, what? We'll translate.

In the fitness world, a pyramid system progresses from using lighter weights and moves up to heavier ones. By contrast, a reverse pyramid system is the opposite—you start with the heaviest weights first and work your way down to the lightest. Both approaches are popular in the weight-training and bodybuilding worlds, but Jen, who designed the workouts that follow, prefers the reverse pyramid system because it's logical: as you do a strength-training workout, you'll get more and more fatigued, so why would you lift the heaviest weights last?

With the modified reverse pyramid format, each circuit is a different length of time, which naturally changes the number of reps you do. (Just so we're clear about the lingo, a *circuit* is a series of exercises that's designed to be completed one after another in quick succession; once you perform all the exercises, you have completed the circuit and can start again.) With the reverse pyramid approach, you'll be doing the heavy lifting at the beginning—when you'll be doing more reps over a longer period of time—then working your way down to a shorter set. We're also calling it a *modified reverse pyramid* because this system uses time, instead of dumbbell weight, to work your way down the pyramid. In addition to helping you avoid getting overly fatigued by the time your biggest set comes around, this approach helps you stay motivated psychologically: since you know you'll be doing fewer reps over a shorter span of time, you feel confident that you can see it through.

But you'll still be pushing your muscles hard, working them to their full capacity over the course of the circuit. And because these circuits include variety in terms of the duration of each segment and hence the number of reps, you'll be helping to change your body composition, losing body fat, and increasing lean muscle mass.

You may have heard that if you keep exposing your body to the same stresses—in this case, the stress of doing resistance exercises—it will adapt to them and stop responding. Say you've never done push-ups before and you decide to do 10 one day; the next day, your arms and chest will feel sore because you will have challenged your muscles and caused tiny tears in their fibers, which is what causes the pain. But if you start doing 10 push-ups every day, you won't experience that muscle soreness anymore because your body will have adapted to the challenge. That's a good thing (because it means you've made progress, plus you'll be pain-free) but also a not-so-good thing (because your muscles won't continue to get stronger from the work).

To reap more benefits, you'll need to increase the number of reps you do or change the style of push-ups you do (from a regular to a wide stance, for example) to challenge your muscles once again. You want to keep your body guessing all the time. One of the best ways to do that is to switch up the length of time you do any given move.

"EPOC" Gains

There's another benefit of this method: by building lean muscle mass, you'll boost your resting metabolic rate, causing your body to burn calories at a higher rate, both after the workout itself as well as throughout the rest of the day and night. The post-workout benefit is called "the afterburn effect"—the technical term is *excess postexercise oxygen consumption,* or EPOC for short—and it causes your body to burn calories at a faster rate for hours after the workout. Each pound of muscle you have uses 6 to 8 calories a day just to sustain itself, whereas every pound of fat burns only 2 calories daily. This means you're burning more calories per day even when you're just sitting on the couch, watching *Amazing Race* shows (as Jen does). This can help you lose weight or at least body fat (but only if you don't compensate by eating more).

One Tough Mother!

To gain the best results for the long term, you'll want to combine intensity and variety for a true one-two punch. Not only will the following workouts get you in the best shape of your life, but because they blend strength-training and cardio intervals, they'll help you train for intense competitions like Tough Mudders and the Spartan Races because they never let your body fully rest. (You can do that later!) These workouts will target the muscles you'll need for these events, helping you build strength and endurance. If these newfangled competitive events, many of which are designed to push you to your limits (and maybe beyond), appeal to you, fine, go for it. Our workouts will set the stage and get you in the right shape so that you can! But these are functional movements, so they'll serve you well in everyday life, too.

Ideally, you'll want to do the program five days per week (they don't have to be consecutive days, but for the sake of simplicity, we've framed the following workouts with a Monday through Friday format); if you're recovering from an injury or you're just getting started, you may want to start with three days a week and add a day per week as you get stronger until you reach a max of five. Avoid doing the program every day so you can give your body some time to rest, which is a vital part of your

Not sure how to do the warm-up moves? Don't sweat it. Use the following descriptions as your guide. Remember that the goal here is to raise your body temperature, warm up your muscles, and enhance your range of motion, not to fully launch your workout.

JUMPING JACK. Stand with your feet together and your arms hanging at your sides. Jump your legs out to a wide stance while lifting your arms up so they're on either side of your head. (Your body will be in an X shape.) As you jump again, move your arms back down to your sides and your legs back in so your feet are together again. Repeat.

SQUAT. Stand with your feet hip-width apart, your arms hanging at your sides or in front of you. Engage your core, bend your knees at a 90-degree angle, and, keeping your chest lifted and the weight in the heels of your feet, lower your body into a squat. Don't let your knees extend beyond your toes. The hip motion should be the same as if you were going to sit on a chair. Push yourself up into a standing position. Repeat.

SHOULDER CROSSOVER. Stand with your feet shoulder-width apart and extend your arms straight out to your sides. Bring them straight in front of your chest, bend your arms, and wrap them around your body (as if you were going to hug yourself), then open them wide and extend them out to the side again. Repeat.

BUTT KICK. Stand with your feet shoulder-width apart then jog in place, kicking your legs up behind you so that your heels touch your butt. Keep moving continuously.

fitness regimen. Your body needs an occasional break to recover, repair its muscles, and replenish its energy; days off will do this for you. If you have a special event to go to and you want to feel like you're at the top of your game (in terms of conditioning), you could do two workouts in a day, perhaps a 30-minute jog in the morning and one of our circuit workouts (or a 20-minute HIIT workout, as outlined in chapter 10) in the afternoon. This way, you'll get double the benefit from the afterburn effect and can burn more calories and body fat to help you slim down faster.

CROSS BODY KICK. Stand with your feet hip-width apart and your feet parallel but your right foot 12 to 18 inches ahead of your left. Extend your right arm straight in front of you, with your hand extended. Kick your left leg up and forward, crossing the midline of your body until it touches your extended right hand. Switch legs (and hands).

ALTERNATING REVERSE LUNGES WITH ROTATION. Stand with your feet shoulder-width apart and step back with your right foot, bending both knees at a 90-degree angle into a reverse lunge. As you lunge, rotate your body toward your front (left) knee, rotating from the waist without twisting either knee. Push up into a standing position, rotate back to center, and repeat with the other leg.

LATERAL LUNGE WITH ALTERNATING TOE TAP. Stand with your feet shoulder-width apart and step out to the side with your right foot, bending into a lateral lunge. As you lunge, keep your chest lifted and reach your left hand across your body to touch the outside of your right foot (or shin if you can't reach the foot). Come back to a standing position, and repeat on the other side.

WALK-OUT TO PLANK. Stand tall with your feet hip-width apart. Bend over so that your hands are touching the floor in front of you, and walk yourself out into a plank position. Your abs should be engaged and your body should be in a straight line. Do a push-up. (If you are new to exercise, you can do a push-up on your knees.) Then, walk your hands back toward your feet and stand up. Repeat.

The **4-3-2-1** Power Grid

Each of the following workouts has four circuits; they are broken down like this:

- 4: Four exercises, each of which should be performed for 60 seconds.
- 3: Three exercises, each of which should be done for 50 seconds.
- 2: Two exercises, each of which should be performed for 40 seconds.
- 1: One exercise that should be performed for 30 seconds.

In other words, each workout follows a 4-3-2-1 pattern; the specific exercises for each are described in detail in other chapters (see the index for exercises you're not familiar with). The circuits are designed to be as efficient and effective as possible, given the time constraints we all live with. You will start with a 3- to 5-minute dynamic warm-up routine to elevate your heart rate and body temperature. Then the four circuits in the actual workout will take you about 12 minutes total, including a 30-second break (start with 45 seconds if you're new to exercise) after each circuit. Repeat all four circuits three times, and follow that with a 3- to 5-minute cool-down stretch for a workout that can be done in 45 minutes or less. If you're totally pressed for time, do the circuit two times instead of three, and you'll still get great benefits. (*Note:* It's a good idea to wear a heart-rate monitor to make sure you're working out hard enough to get the results you want.)

Warm-Up

Perform each of the following moves for 30 seconds each:

Jumping Jack

Squat

Shoulder Crossover

Butt Kick

Cross Body Kick

Alternating Reverse Lunge with Rotation

Lateral Lunge with Alternating Toe Tap

Walk-Out to Plank

The **4-3-2-1** Circuit Workouts

You can always mix and match the exercises and increase and decrease the weight of the dumbbell(s) you're using. With this approach, you will never plateau because you'll be subjecting your body to constant change! The 30-second resting periods between circuits are important because they allow time for your heart rate to come back down after going up. This up-and-down pattern produces maximum cardiovascular effects and triggers the (metabolic) fat-burning process.

WEEK 1

Monday

Deep Squat with Overhead Rotation

Side Plank with Forward Arm Extension
(30 seconds to each side)

Incline Chest Press in Wall Squat

Curtsy Lunge with Dumbbells

Alternating-Arm Chest Press

Basic Plank

Basic Push-Up

Tabletop with Elbow-to-Knee Crunch (right side)

Tabletop with Elbow-to-Knee Crunch (left side)

Deadlift

Tuesday

4

Alternating Lunge

Standing W-press

Bent-Over Rear Fly

Mountain Climber

3

Extended-Arm Bicep Curl with Knee Raise

Hammer Curl

Squat with Overhead Press

2

Ball Crunch (a basic crunch with your back on a stability ball; as you progress, you can do alternating leg extensions as you crunch)

Superman

1

Russian Twist

Wednesday

Walk-Out to Push-Up

Skull Crusher on a Stability Ball

Lateral Lunge with Dumbbell (right side)

Lateral Lunge with Dumbbell (left side)

Triceps Tower

Forward Lunge with Woodchopper (right side)

Forward Lunge with Woodchopper (left side)

Side V-ups (right side)

Side V-ups (left side)

Lateral Step-Out Squats

Thursday

4

Inverted Row

Alternating Big Row

Bicep-Shoulder Combo (30 seconds on one side then switch sides)

Plank Jack

3

Fast Feet

Deadlift with Rotation Twist

Hamstring Pull-In with Ball

2

Curtsy Lunge with alternate arm extension

Dumbbell Swing

1

Stability Ball Roll-In

Friday

 4

Reverse Lunge with Kick (right leg)

Reverse Lunge with Kick (left leg)

Lateral Lunge with Half X (right side)

Lateral Lunge with Half X (left side)

 3

Lateral Raise

Step-Up

Ballet Arms

 2

Side-to-Side Push-Up

Grapple Throw

 1

Plank with Alternating Knee-to-Elbow Rotations

WEEK 2

Monday

 Side Step to Side Kick on sturdy chair or platform (right side)

Side Step to Side Kick on sturdy chair or platform (left side)

Arnold Press on chair or stability ball

Body Roll-Out

 Half Jack with Dumbbells

Bent-Over Wide Row

Plank to Row

 Vertical Leap

Rotator Cuff Raise (a.k.a. the Scarecrow)

 Inverted Row

Tuesday

4

Single-Leg Deadlift (right side)

Single-Leg Deadlift (left side)

Tabletop with Elbow-to-Knee Crunch (right side)

Tabletop with Elbow-to-Knee Crunch (left side)

3

Hamstring Pull-In with Ball

Alternating Cross-Leg Push-Up

Squat with Overhead Press

2

Jump Squat

Staggered Push-Up (switch hand position halfway through)

1

Back Extension on a Ball

Wednesday

 Offset Squat (right side)

Offset Squat (left side)

Offset Split Lunge with Shoulder Press (right side)

Offset Split Lunge with Shoulder Press (left side)

 Inverted Row

Bent-Over Wide Row

Swimmer

 Vertical Sit-Up with Crossover Elbow to Knee (right side)

Vertical Sit-Up with Crossover Elbow to Knee (left side)

 Plank Drag with Towel

Thursday

4
Plié with Upright Row

Single-Leg Squat (right leg)

Single-Leg Squat (left leg)

Alternating Cross Leg Push-Up

3
Burpee

Side Plank with Triceps Extension (right side)

Side Plank with Triceps Extension (left side)

2
Side V-up (right side)

Side V-up (left side)

1
Jump Lunge

Friday

 4

Reverse Leg Press (right side)

Reverse Leg Press (left side)

Forward Lunge with Woodchopper (right leg)

Forward Lunge with Woodchopper (left leg)

 3

In-Out Bicep Curl

Bent-Over Wide Row

Dumbbell Pullover (on the floor, or use a stability ball for more intensity and core work)

 2

In and Out

180-Degree Jump

 1

Russian Twist

WEEK 3

Monday

Squat Thrust

Decline Push-Up

Reverse Dumbbell Press (on the floor, or use a stability ball to crank up the core intensity)

Sumo Squat Jump

Single-Leg Deadlift (right leg)

Single-Leg Deadlift (left leg)

Grapple Throw

Single-Arm Chest Press (right side)

Single-Arm Chest Press (left side)

Push-Up to a T (alternate sides)

Tuesday

 4
Lateral Lunge with Knee-to-Elbow Rotation (right leg)

Lateral Lunge with Knee-to-Elbow Rotation (left leg)

Wide Push-Up

Box Jump

 3
Back Extensions on a Ball

Bent-Over Rear Fly

Suicide Row

 2
Side Plank with Triceps Extension (right side)

Side Plank with Triceps Extension (left side)

 1
Triceps Dip (on a stability ball)

Wednesday

 4

One-Legged Glute Bridge (30 seconds on each leg)

Curtsy Lunges (alternating sides)

Rotator-Cuff Raise (a.k.a. the Scarecrow)

Half Jack with Dumbbells

 3

Superman

Bulgarian Lunge (right side)

Bulgarian Lunge (left side)

 2

Staggered Push-Up (change hand positions halfway through)

Hamstring Pull-In with Ball

 1

Side-to-Side Ball Crunch

Thursday

 4
- Deep Squat with Overhead Rotation
- Plié with Upward Row
- Front Lunge with Dumbbell Pass-Through (right side)
- Front Lunge with Dumbbell Pass-Through (left side)

 3
- Shoulder Windmill with Plié
- Windmill with Dumbbell (right side)
- Windmill with Dumbbell (left side)

 2
- Bicep-Shoulder Combo
- Hammer Curl

 1
- Reverse Tabletop

Friday

Single-Leg Squat (right leg)

Single-Leg Squat (left leg)

In and Out

Reverse Dumbbell Press

Reverse Leg Press (Right Side)

Reverse Leg Press (Left Side)

Push-Up to T

Vertical Leap

Pendulum Jump

Spider-Man Plank Crunch

KEEPING IT FRESH

At first blush, figuring out how to include variety in a strength-training routine may seem hard. But with 642 skeletal muscles in the human body, you certainly can mix up your strength-training regimen to keep it lively and interesting. Switch up the variables at least every two or three months, and try the following approaches because each one provides different benefits. Variety really is the spice of progress! Here are twenty ways to get it.

SPLITS

We're not talking about the kinds of splits that are done in gymnastics. We're talking about body-part splits—which muscles you will hit in each workout. You can mix up how you split your training in the following ways:

1. **The Full-Body Approach.** This style hits all the major muscle groups in the legs, back, chest, shoulders, and abdomen in a single workout. This setup will strengthen each muscle group effectively if you use it for one out of three workouts per week.
2. **The Push/Pull Split.** This approach divides the body into muscles that go through a pushing motion (such as the quadriceps, chest, triceps, and fronts of the shoulders) versus muscles that go through pulling motions (such as the hamstrings, back muscles, biceps, and rear deltoids). The idea is that you'll work only the push muscles on one day and only the pull muscles on a separate day. This way, each muscle group receives a more focused workout once or twice per week.
3. **The Upper/Lower Split.** With this one, you switch between workouts that focus solely on the upper body then solely on the lower body in alternate workouts. As with the Push/Pull Split, this approach gives each muscle group a more focused workout once or twice per week.

4. **The Body-Part Split.** Each workout focuses solely on one or two body parts at a time. For example, your chest, back, arm, leg, and abdominal muscles would all be addressed on separate days. This method works each muscle group once a week at a higher intensity.

PATTERNS OF EXERCISES

After deciding which workout split you want to use, you have another choice to make: how would you like to handle the pattern for the individual workouts? Here are your options:

5. **Straight Sets.** Complete all the sets of each exercise one at a time before moving on to the next exercise. This is a great approach when you're aiming for a hard-core workout.

6. **Super Sets.** Complete two exercises back to back with minimal rest (30 to 60 seconds) between sets. Finish all sets of each group before moving on to the next group of exercises.

7. **Circuit Training.** Do one set of each exercise in the circuit in a sequential fashion, with little to no rest between the moves. Rest for a minute or two after completing all the exercises, then go through the circuit again, rest (briefly) again, then take one more pass through the circuit. This is a wonderful way to fit cardio and weight training into one workout.

TYPES OF EXERCISES

You can also structure your workouts, according to the types of exercises involved. Here are some ways to do that:

8. **The Basics.** This includes moves like squats, rows, deadlifts, bench presses, and the like—classic moves that have been around forever because they work. Don't shy away from them.

9. **Body Weight Exercises.** These rely on your own body weight to provide resistance. But just because a move doesn't involve equipment doesn't mean it's a cinch to do. These exercises (push-ups, planks, and the like) challenge the body effectively—and they can be done anywhere, which is a real bonus!

10. **Stabilization Exercises.** Adding a component of stability and balance to an exercise provides an extra challenge and forces the muscles to work in new, more functional ways. These exercises include things like one-legged squats or one-handed triceps dips.

11. **Plyometric Exercises.** Adding a few high-intensity, explosive moves (like burpees, vertical leaps, and lateral jumps) to a workout not only increases your heart rate but also helps you build power and lean muscle.

12. **Compound Exercises.** These moves (such as a lunge–bicep curl–shoulder press combo) challenge more than one body part at a time and can help make effective use of your workout time. Plus, they often require more stabilization.

13. **Functional Exercises.** Moves like a squat to an overhead press or a side lunge with rotation mimic everyday activities or a common range of motion in a specific sport or activity. They help to build strength, stability, and endurance where you need these elements the most.

REP SCHEMES

You can also play with the number of reps you do for individual exercises. This will help keep your muscles guessing, which will help them build strength faster. There are different ways to do this:

14. **Lower Reps.** Sticking with 8 or fewer reps with a heavier weight challenges your strength, but don't worry: you will *not* bulk up! Instead, you will turbocharge your metabolism and add more muscle definition.

15. **Moderate Reps**. Staying in the 8 to 12 range for reps, with moderately heavy weights, increases strength and endurance. This rep range is a great solid base for a general workout.

16. **Higher Reps.** You can build up muscle endurance using slightly lighter weights and by doing 15 or more reps at a time. This way, your muscles spend more time under pressure.

17. **Pyramids.** You can increase or decrease the number of reps that you complete in each set (as we do with our circuit workouts). For example, you might start with 15 reps on the first set, then drop down to 12 on the second set, 10 on the third, and 6 on the fourth, while increasing the amount of weight you're lifting with each set. Or you could start low on the number of reps and work your way up.

18. **Drop Sets.** Instead of ending a set when you reach the point of fatigue, lower the amount of weight you're using in the exercise by about 10 percent and continue to do as many reps as possible with the lighter weight. Drop the amount of weight a second or third time if necessary to reach maximum muscle fatigue.

19. **Timed Sets.** Instead of aiming for a certain number of reps, set a timer and complete as many reps as you can (with stellar form!) for the allotted time.

20. **Tempo Sets.** Do a lower number of reps but use a tempo that's much slower than normal or hold the weight for a few counts in the middle of the movement (for example, at the bottom of a squat).

Cool It—By Stretching It Out

After completing the circuit workout, take a few minutes to stretch. It's a great way to cool down, slow your heart rate, and enhance the flexibility of your muscles and the range of motion in your joints. There are different schools of thought on stretching. Our feeling is that static stretching—which involves a slow, controlled elongation of a muscle for 15 to 30 seconds—is the best way to go after a workout. You should always stretch the tightest muscles first (like the hip flexors, which we rely on constantly in everyday life—for walking, sitting, climbing stairs, and more), since the tighter muscles will usually inhibit the stretch of your other muscles. And you should always stretch to the point of gentle tension, but not pain!

Here are the key ones to include:

CROSS-SHOULDER STRETCH. Stand with your feet hip-width apart and your knees slightly bent. Keep your shoulders level, bend your right elbow, and extend your right arm across your chest; place your left hand on your right elbow to gently support your arm during the stretch. Hold it for 10 to 15 seconds, then release. Repeat with the left arm.

CHEST STRETCH. Stand with your feet hip-width apart and your knees slightly bent. Keep your shoulders level and place your arms behind your back, clasping your hands together. Extend your arms straight behind you. Hold for 10 to 15 seconds, feeling the stretch in your chest, then release.

BICEP STRETCH. Stand with your feet hip-width apart and a slight bend in your knees. Keep your shoulders down and extend your right arm out in front of you with your palm facing up, and bend your fingers back slightly with your left hand. You should feel a gentle stretch in your right forearm and bicep muscles. Hold for 10 to 15 seconds, then release. Repeat with the left arm.

OVERHEAD TRICEPS STRETCH. Stand with your feet hip-width apart and a slight bend in your knees. Keep your shoulders down and bend your right elbow as you lift your right arm up next to your head. Place the fingers of your right hand

ROPE CLIMBS

With this challenge, you'll want to use your legs to get up the rope, rather than depending solely on upper-body strength (as many people do). Jump up to grab the rope high, gripping it tightly with both hands. Let the rope fall on the outside of one leg and wrap the rope over the top of that foot, looping it under the other foot, at the arch. Bring your knees up to your chest, let the rope slide down below your feet and use both feet to pinch the rope, thus locking it in place and anchoring yourself. Stand on the rope to gain more height as you once again reach up with your hands as high as possible and grip the rope higher up. Release the rope from your feet and use your abs to bring your knees to your chest as you re-secure your feet on the rope, pinching it tightly. Continue this inchworm technique until you reach the top. If you can't make it to the top on your first try, don't sweat it; aim for the halfway point or even a third of the way up and add to your distance as your strength and comfort levels increase.

behind your head so they touch the shoulder blade area. Meanwhile, place your left arm over the top of your head and your left hand on your right elbow to gently support your right arm during the stretch. Hold for 10 to 15 seconds, then release. Repeat with the left arm.

QUAD STRETCH. Stand and face a wall, leaving about a foot's distance, and place your left hand against it for balance. Raise your right foot behind you (toward your butt) and grab your right foot with your right hand. Keep your knees parallel as you gently pull your right heel up toward your bottom, stretching the muscles in the front of your right thigh. Hold for 15 to 20 seconds then release. Repeat on the other side.

GROIN STRETCH. Sit on the floor with your feet together, sole to sole, and your knees opened to the sides (butterfly style). Place your elbows on the inside of your knees and slowly push down until you feel a stretch along the insides of your thighs. Hold the stretch for 10 to 15 seconds, then release. Repeat.

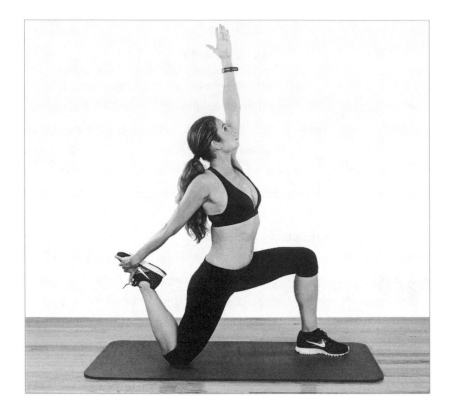

HIP FLEXOR STRETCH. Kneel on your right knee with your toes facing the floor, and place your left foot flat on the floor in front of you, your left knee bent at a 90-degree angle. Gently press your hips forward until you feel tension in the front of your right thigh. For a more intense stretch, try grabbing your back (left) foot and extending the other (right) arm toward the ceiling. Hold the stretch for 15 seconds then release. Switch sides.

HAMSTRING STRETCH. Lie on your back with both knees bent. Place your feet flat on the floor, about 6 inches apart, and bring your right knee up toward your chest, holding the back of your right leg with both hands behind your calf. Slowly straighten your right leg until you feel the stretch in the back of your leg. Hold the stretch for 15 to 20 seconds then release. Repeat with the left leg.

TOE-TOUCH STRETCH. While sitting on the floor, extend both legs straight out in front of you and flex your feet. Reach your fingertips toward your feet as far as you can go. Hold this position for 15 seconds, then release.

10

Torching the Fat

Getting stronger and fitter is really a two-step process: you need to do strength-training to build lean muscle mass, and you need to do the right forms of cardio-vascular exercise to burn body fat. This dynamic duo will deliver the get-strong, get-sexy results you want faster than any other approach (assuming you also stick with a healthy, clean eating plan). The good news is that the cardio part of the equation doesn't have to take over your life. You can put time on your side with high-intensity interval training (HIIT, for short), a smoking-hot cardiorespiratory training technique that alternates bouts of speed work and recovery to crank up the overall intensity of your workout; Tabata, Insanity, and CrossFit are among the most popular HIIT-style workouts. HIIT is one of the best ways to spice up a mundane cardio workout and pack a huge metabolism-boosting punch in a short amount of time.

The HIIT approach also carries a whole bunch of specific health benefits. Research has found that it delivers a significant boost in aerobic (cardiorespiratory) fitness and anaerobic (muscle-strengthening) fitness, reduces belly and overall body fat, lowers fasting insulin, and increases insulin sensitivity (a combo that can reduce your risk of developing type 2 diabetes), boosts metabolism (which can help with weight loss), improves HDL (the "good") cholesterol, reduces blood pressure, and improves blood levels of health-protecting antioxidants. What's more, HIIT increased cardiorespiratory function nearly twofold over moderate-intensity continuous training among people with heart-related diseases, according to a recent review of studies on the subject by researchers at the University of Queensland in Australia. So you have nothing to lose and so much to gain from HIIT-ing it.

By alternating short bouts of high-intensity exercise with recovery intervals, HIIT gives you a huge bang for your exercise efforts, and it can be a fun change of pace from what you may now be doing. While most endurance workouts (like running or walking) are done at a moderate intensity (and often at a steady pace), high-intensity intervals are performed at an exertion level of 7 to 9 (on a scale of 1 to 10, with 1 being no effort and 10 being as hard as you can possibly push yourself) for anywhere from 30 seconds to 3 minutes at a time. In between, there are recovery intervals (anywhere from 10 seconds to 5 minutes) that allow you to catch your breath, recoup your energy, and get ready for the next burst of intensity. Sessions typically last from 9 to no more than 30 minutes and incorporate fast-paced, challenging strength-building, cardio-pumping moves like squats, squat jumps, side-to-side shuffle jumps, burpees, mountain climbers, and the like. (If you don't know what some of these moves are, don't worry. You'll find out in this book!)

Best of all, these short-duration, high-intensity sessions can crank up the cardio benefits, build muscle strength and endurance, and torch body fat and calories. One of the main principles behind these workouts is to avoid steady-state exercise, which your body can adapt to quickly, so HIIT workouts challenge your body to adjust to continuously changing moves, which builds faster fitness results. Another boon: HIIT will help you avoid slamming up against an exercise plateau.

As you get stronger and fitter, you'll notice that the workouts you've been doing have gotten easier. That's a good thing—and a bad thing, too. The good part means that you've made lots of progress; it means that what used to be challenging for your body is no big deal now. The bad part means that your muscles, lungs, heart, and other body parts have adapted to the moves, and you are no longer getting as much out of them in terms of cardio-boosting, strength-building, or calorie-burning benefits. This also means that you need to take your workouts to the next level or else you'll end up on an exercise plateau (stuck, in other words!), and it will become difficult to improve your fitness condition further, even if you're already fairly fit. The key, then, is to shock your body by introducing more intense segments to your workouts, to essentially jump-start your body's fitness gains once again. Doing HIIT training with one type of exercise can even have a positive ripple effect on other forms: a recent study from Loughborough University in the United Kingdom found that when triathletes did six sessions of high-intensity cycle interval training over three weeks, they experienced improvements in both their cycling and running performance.

And because the duration of HIIT workouts is short and the moves progress so quickly, the whole thing is over before you know it. That may be why it appeals to those who love exercise (because it's challenging) as well as those who don't (because the time passes so fast). By the way, HIIT is a great way to train for those super hard-core, newfangled races that are all the rage these days (like the Spartan Race or Tough Mudders of the world). It's time, then, to give the HIIT approach a try—and take your *Strong Is the New Skinny* program to the next level. Here are three HIIT workouts you can do at home, without any equipment (just your body!). You'll want to use your smartphone or a stopwatch to time your intervals. If you're a beginner, use a smaller range of motion or lighter weights with each of these and build up gradually.

The Exercises Deconstructed

You've already learned how to do many of these HIIT exercises in other chapters. (Review those descriptions if you need to.) But for those that are new, here's your decoder ring:

180-Degree Jump

Get into a squat position with your body weight in your heels and your knees in line with your toes. From here jump up and turn 180 degrees until you're facing the opposite direction. (*Note:* You can swing your arms to propel yourself along.)

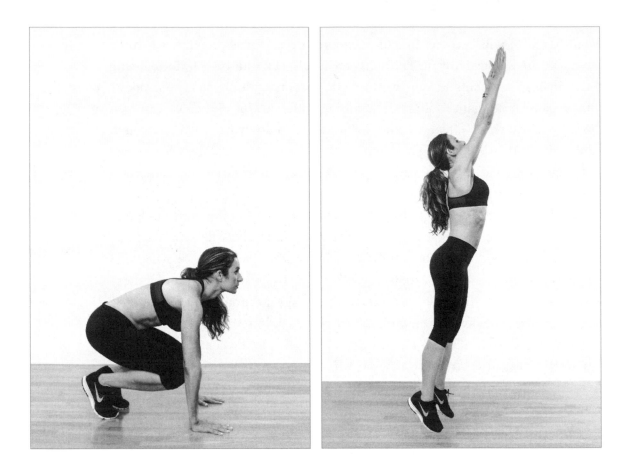

Burpee

Assume a push-up position, then pull your legs in toward your chest so your feet land near your hands. Jump up in the air while raising your arms above your head.

Side-to-Side Core Rotation

Stand with your feet shoulder-width apart and hold one dumbbell in both hands (one end in each hand). Rotate the dumbbell to your right side, then your left side, continuing back and forth while keeping your hips facing forward; in other words, rotate from the waist rather than the hips.

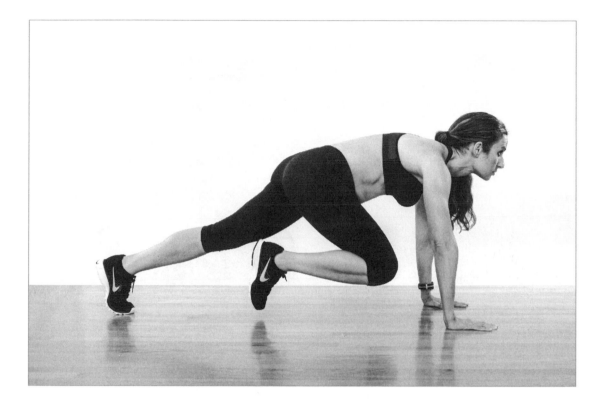

Mountain Climber

Assume a push-up position with your hands under your shoulders and your feet hip-width apart. Lift your right foot and bend your knee in toward your chest, then return it to the starting position as you simultaneously bring your left knee in toward your chest. Alternate legs and keep your pace as fast as possible so that you're essentially jumping your feet in and out; keep your butt low and in line with your torso throughout the move.

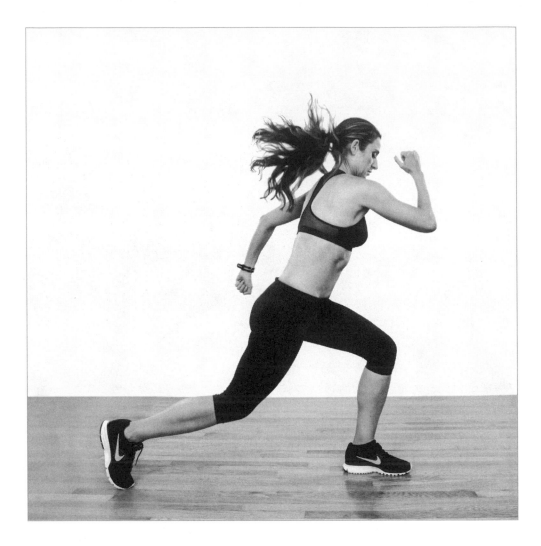

Jump Lunge

Stand with your feet shoulder-width apart and step forward onto your right foot into a lunge position; your left leg should be straight out behind you with your foot flexed and on the ground. Lower yourself into a lunge with both knees bent at 90-degree angles. From here, explode out of your lunge into a jump, straightening both legs. As you land, lower yourself back into another lunge on your right foot. Work on the right side, and then switch to your left.

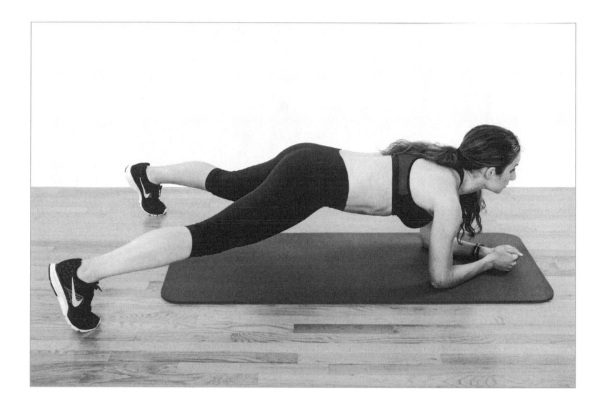

Plank Jack

Get into a plank position with your forearms on the floor, shoulders and elbows in line, legs long, and feet together. Your core should be engaged, and your body should stay in a straight line. Jump your feet out wide (just as you do with a regular jumping jack), then in again to the starting position. Your body should remain low and parallel to the ground.

Fast Feet

Stand in a wide stance with your knees bent slightly. Jog in place as quickly as possible, picking up and putting down your feet at a rapid pace. You only need to lift your feet a couple of inches off the ground before putting them back down. Keep your body low, and try not to bounce up and down.

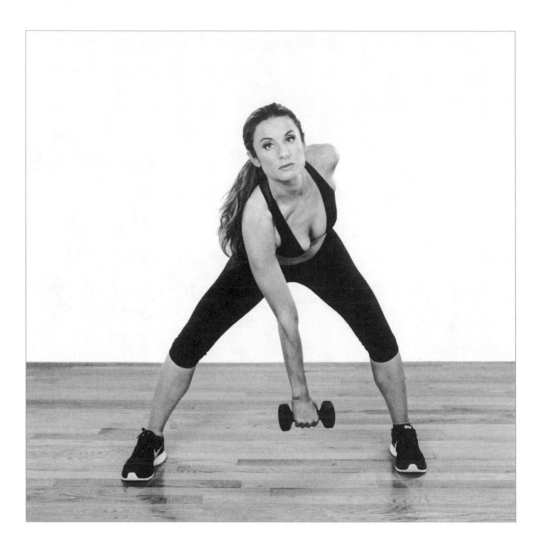

Half Jack with Dumbbells

Hold a dumbbell in each hand by your hips. Do a jumping jack with your feet and extend one dumbbell down toward the floor and the other one behind your back; return to the upright position with the dumbbells by your hips. Then, do another jumping jack and bring the opposite dumbbell down toward the floor; return to the starting position. Continue this pattern at a steady pace.

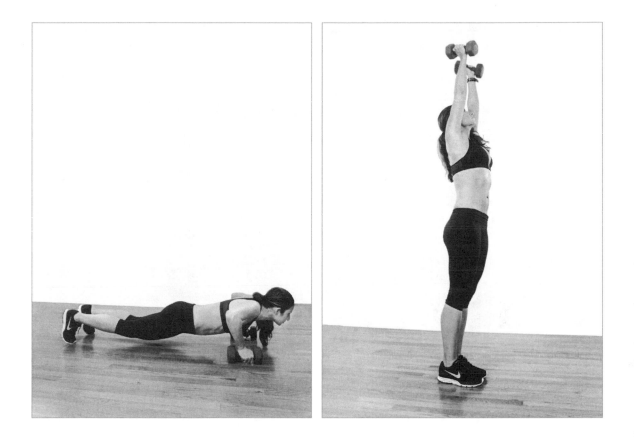

Suicide Row

This move sounds scary, but it's really not, and it's worth it because it gives you cardio and strength training at the same time! Start in a plank position with your feet hip-width apart and hold a dumbbell in each hand under your shoulders. Make sure your abs are engaged to keep your body in a tight, straight line. Do a push-up by lowering yourself toward the ground until your arms are bent at 90-degree angles and then extending and straightening your arms. When you reach the top of the extension, lift the right dumbbell, driving your right elbow up and back in a "row," keeping your arm close to your body. Return the right dumbbell to the floor and resume the plank position; do a push-up then a row on your left side. (*Note:* If you're having a hard time balancing, you can widen your stance for more support.) After doing a row on each side, jump your feet toward your hands and stand up, pressing the dumbbells over your head toward the ceiling when you're standing. Then bring your arms back down to your sides and repeat the sequence.

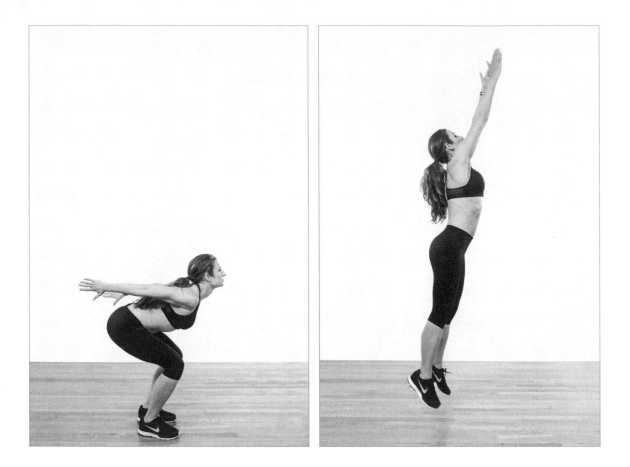

Vertical Leap

Stand with your feet shoulder-width apart and your arms at your sides. Bend your knees and hinge forward from your waist, thrusting your hips forward as you jump straight up into the air. You can swing your arms up for momentum (you're going up and down as high as you can, without moving forward or back). Return to standing.

Squat Thrust

Stand with your feet shoulder-width apart. Bend your knees until your hands can touch the ground on either side of your feet; your butt should be tucked down toward the ground. From here, kick your legs behind you so they land in a push-up position. Next jump your feet back into your squatting position and stand up. Repeat.

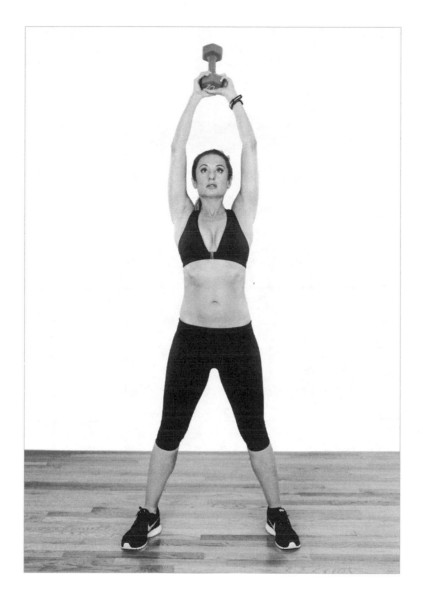

Dumbbell Swing

Start in a squatting position with your feet hip-width apart and your toes pointing forward. Hold a dumbbell in both hands down between your legs. While keeping your arms straight and the weight clasped firmly, swing the dumbbell up over your head in a controlled motion, pushing yourself into a standing position on the upswing. In a fluid motion, lower the dumbbell back down and return to your squat starting position.

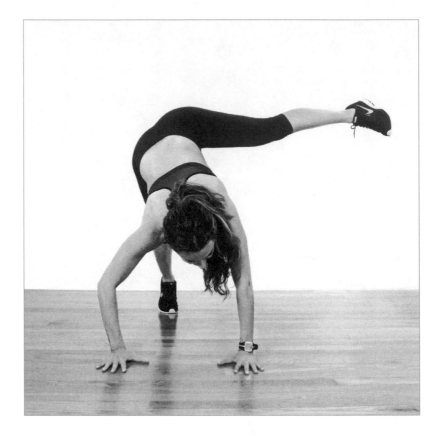

Pendulum Jump

With your feet in a wide stance, hinge forward from your waist and place your hands on the floor in front of you. Extend your right leg straight out to the side; your left (supporting) leg can be slightly bent. From this position, quickly transfer your body weight to the other (right) leg while the supporting (left) leg extends out to the side. Keep doing this back and forth at a steady pace. Your hands should never leave the ground.

High Knees

Stand tall with your feet shoulder-width apart and your arms straight out in front at waist height; your palms should be facing the floor. Jog in place, driving one knee then the other up to a 90-degree angle so they meet your hands. Try to go as quickly as you can. Make sure to keep your back straight; don't lean forward.

The 10-Minute HIIT

WARM-UP

1 minute: Squats (with your feet parallel and slightly wider than your hips)

1 minute: Alternating Knee-to-Chest Raises

30 seconds: Burpees

15 seconds: Rest by marching (or stepping) in place

30 seconds: 180-Degree Jumps

15 seconds: Rest by marching (or stepping) in place

30 seconds: Mountain Climbers

15 seconds: Rest by marching (or stepping) in place

30 seconds: Jump Lunges

15 seconds: Rest by marching (or stepping) in place

Repeat the sequence once more.

COOLDOWN (MINI CORE WORKOUT)

1 minute: Side-to-Side Squats

1 minute: V-ups

The 20-Minute HIIT

WARM-UP

1 minute: Alternating Reverse Lunges

1 minute: Side-to-Side Core Rotations

1 minute: Jumping Jacks

30 seconds: Mountain Climbers

15 seconds: Rest by marching (or stepping) in place

30 seconds: Sumo Squat Jumps

15 seconds: Rest by marching (or stepping) in place

30 seconds: Spider-Man Plank Crunches

15 seconds: Rest by marching (or stepping) in place

30 seconds: Fast Feet

15 seconds: Rest by marching (or stepping) in place

30 seconds: Curtsy Lunges

15 seconds: Rest by marching (or stepping) in place

Repeat 3 more times.

COOLDOWN (MINI CORE WORKOUT)

1 minute: Lateral Lunges with Knee-to-Elbow Rotation

30 seconds: Side V-ups (right side)

30 seconds: Side V-ups (left side)

The 30-Minute HIIT

WARM-UP

> **1 minute:** Lateral Step-Out Squats
>
> **1 minute:** Walk-Outs to Plank
>
> **1 minute:** Woodchoppers (30 seconds on each leg)

30 seconds: Dumbbell Swing

15 seconds: Rest by marching (or stepping) in place

30 seconds: Plank Jacks

15 seconds: Rest by marching (or stepping) in place

30 seconds: Half Jacks with Dumbbells

15 seconds: Rest by marching (or stepping) in place

30 seconds: Suicide Rows

15 seconds: Rest by marching (or stepping) in place

Repeat the sequence 3 more times and then continue with . . .

30 seconds: 4 High Knees and 4 Plank Jacks

15 seconds: Rest by marching (or stepping) in place

30 seconds: 4 Squat Thrusts and 4 Half Jacks with Dumbbells

15 seconds: Rest by marching (or stepping) in place

30 seconds: 4 Dumbbell Swings and 4 Vertical Leaps

15 seconds: Rest by marching (or stepping) in place

30 seconds: 4 Pendulum Jumps and 4 Box Jumps

15 seconds: Rest by marching (or stepping) in place

Repeat the circuit 3 more times.

COOLDOWN (MINI CORE WORKOUT)

1 minute: Side-to-Side Sumo Squats (This is the same move as regular sumo squats but this time you're stepping out from side to side: lower your hips, then rise with your dumbbell on one side; repeat on the other side.)

1 minute: Russian Twists

1 minute: Vertical Sit-Ups with Crossover Elbow to Knee

WHAT'S YOUR TARGET HEART RATE?

Most people don't have a clue what theirs is. At first blush, it may seem complicated to figure out, but it really isn't. The best way to figure out your target heart rate is by using the Karvonen formula, which factors in your resting heart rate and reflects the training heart rate based on a percentage of your maximum heart rate. (To measure your resting heart rate, take your pulse for 1 full minute first thing in the morning; if you don't feel like counting it for a minute, do it for 30 seconds and multiply it by 2.)

Here's what the formula looks like:

220 – your age = X
X – your resting heart rate = Y
Y × 65 percent (the low end of your aerobic training zone) = A
Y × 85 percent (the high end of your aerobic training zone) = B
Minimum training heart rate = A + resting heart rate
Maximum training heart rate = B + resting heart rate

Based on this formula, here's how a thirty-year-old woman with a resting heart rate of 62 would calculate her training zone:

220 – 30 = 190 (X)
190 – 62 = 128 (Y)
128 × 0.65 = 83.2 (A)
128 × 0.85 = 108.8 (B)
83.2 + 62 = 145.2 (minimum training heart rate)
108.8 + 62 = 170.8 (maximum training heart rate)

As you can see by the last two sums, her target heart rate zone would be 145 to 171 beats per minute.

HOW HARD ARE YOU WORKING?

You know how it's easy to *under*estimate how much you eat? Well, it's also very common for people to *over*estimate how hard they're exercising. Our brains just naturally skew things in our favor in these areas, but this doesn't exactly help us reach our health and fitness goals. That's why it's smart to give yourself a reality check by paying attention to the intensity of your workouts, which also determines the cardiovascular benefits you'll get from them. The easiest way to do this is to wear a heart-rate monitor. These gadgets just don't lie; they tell you exactly how hard you're working based on your heart rate. If it's not in your target zone, you'll know it's time to crank up the intensity of your workout. (By the way, Jen loves her Polar heart-rate monitor because it's simple to use and very accurate.) There's also the *rating of perceived exertion* (RPE) scale, a measure of how hard you feel you're working from 0 (not at all) to 10 (almost your maximum effort). A level 7 or higher is considered a strong intensity; that's what you should aim for with HIIT.

Or, you can use the talk test: If you can chat effortlessly, whistle, or belt out a tune during your workout, your exercise intensity is low. If you can talk with some effort but you're slightly out of breath, you're in the moderate zone. If you can't say more than a few words at a time because your breathing is rapid, you're exercising at a high intensity, which is what you want with HIIT training. So pay attention to these signs of how hard you're really pushing yourself; it'll help you avoid fooling yourself about your exercise intensity.

With the HIIT approach, the harder you go, the better your results will be. Besides, there's no reason to hold back because these workouts are short in duration and varied in their pacing. So right after you get breathless, you'll have a recovery interval before you go hard again. The whole workout will fly by before you know it, and in a matter of weeks you'll get the results that prove the approach is worth the effort.

The HIIT List

There are several different forms of HIIT workouts. While basic aerobic interval training involves relatively long work periods (generally 2 to 5 minutes at a pace that challenges you to make it to the end of that work interval) and shorter rest periods (between 30 and 60 seconds), HIIT workouts crank up the intensity a few notches. Here's how the different HIIT styles stack up.

MAXIMAL HIGH-INTENSITY INTERVAL TRAINING. This type includes intervals that are *very* high intensity (like box jumps, jump lunges, jumping body tucks, or anything else that involves explosive movements), which makes it very effective for burning fat and conditioning your cardiovascular system. You essentially push yourself to the max with every work interval, which is what makes it extremely effective training for sports that require all-out repeated efforts, such as football, soccer, hockey, kickboxing, or sparring.

Maximal intervals are much shorter than aerobic intervals—generally maximal work intervals are 30 seconds or less—whereas rest periods depend largely on the fitness level of the person doing it and/or how much she wants to recover between intervals. Shorter rest periods make the work intervals more challenging, but the pace of the work will also drop quickly after a few intervals. By contrast, longer rest periods allow the body to recover a little more, promoting faster speeds on subsequent intervals. Overall, rest periods should be at least as long as the work periods in order to allow ample recovery so you can perform well during the next work interval.

Since maximal intervals are so challenging, don't expect to be able to jump right in at a high level for a large number of intervals. It's very important to build up gradually. Start by performing five maximal intervals the first two times you do the training; during the next two sessions after that, increase to six maximal intervals. Continue adding intervals in this step-up fashion until you are doing intervals for a maximum of 15 minutes straight. Here's a sample of how to do it.

- **Interval 1:** 30 seconds hard, 30 seconds rest
- **Interval 2:** 30 seconds hard, 30 seconds rest

- **Interval 3:** 25 seconds hard, 30 seconds rest
- **Interval 4:** 25 seconds hard, 30 seconds rest
- **Interval 5:** 20 seconds hard, 30 seconds rest
- **Interval 6:** 20 seconds hard, 30 seconds rest
- **Interval 7:** 15 seconds hard, 30 seconds rest
- **Interval 8:** 15 seconds hard, 30 seconds rest

SUBMAXIMAL HIGH-INTENSITY INTERVALS. This style, outlined below, is excellent for building up your cardiovascular conditioning. It's similar in concept and execution to the maximal interval style. The difference is, instead of pushing yourself as hard as you can (a.k.a. to the max) during each work interval, you work at a pace that is somewhat below your maximum effort. This allows you to do more total work intervals during the session while still keeping your intensity levels high. Most interval programs on cardio machines (like the treadmill or elliptical) follow this principle: the resistance and/or speed are increased to a higher level for a set period of time, then reduced for a set period of time. The level is not so high that you must put your maximum effort into each work interval, but it is at a level that you could not sustain for long periods.

This type of training is also very effective for burning fat and increasing your metabolism. The intervals in this style can be longer than with the maximal high-intensity interval training, since you're not working at your maximum effort, but they're not longer by much. Generally, work and rest periods are 30 to 60 seconds each. Here are some sample intervals you can use in your training.

- **Interval 1:** 30 seconds work, 30 seconds rest
- **Interval 2:** 30 seconds work, 1 minute rest
- **Interval 3:** 1 minute work, 1 minute rest
- **Interval 4:** 1 minute work, 30 seconds rest
- **Interval 5:** 45 seconds work, 45 seconds rest

This type of training can be done for 15 to 30 minutes at a time, depending on the intensity level of the work being performed.

NEAR-MAXIMAL AEROBIC INTERVALS. A unique form of interval training, this style basically combines aerobic interval training with maximal interval training to allow you to work at near-peak levels for long periods of time. This has the benefit of burning a tremendous amount of calories for a longer duration than is possible with regular intervals. While the work intervals themselves are short, the rest periods are much shorter. Instead of pushing yourself to the max on every interval, you work at a pace somewhat short of your max, which allows you to perform near your max for longer periods of time.

This type of training works well with cardio machines that allow you to switch resistance very quickly (such as stationary bikes, stair machines, or elliptical trainers) but not with machines that cycle slowly through their speed adjustments (treadmills fall into this category). It can also be done with running then walking, cycling then pedaling slowly, or even swimming hard then stroking lazily. You'll find it very challenging to have to constantly restart your momentum on every interval.

Here are some sample intervals you can use in your training.

- **Interval 1:** 20 seconds work, 5 seconds rest
- **Interval 2:** 25 seconds work, 5 seconds rest
- **Interval 3:** 30 seconds work, 10 seconds rest
- **Interval 4:** 15 seconds work, 7 seconds rest
- **Interval 5:** 40 seconds work, 10 seconds rest

Continue repeating this cycle for the duration of your HIIT workout (whether it's 5 minutes, 10 minutes, 15 minutes, or up to 30 minutes max).

NOTE: With any of these, it's a mistake to stop what you're doing entirely during your rest period. Keep moving even if you're moving very slowly.

Conclusion

Becoming Your Strongest, Sexiest Self

Hopefully, you've already started having a kinder, more supportive, more empowered conversation with your body, and you've started treating, feeding, and moving it in healthier ways. Maybe you've even begun to discover and embrace what your body can do, beyond just how it looks, and found ways to maximize your physique's strength and power in everyday life. *Kudos!* You've made a committed decision to change your daily routine, whatever it has been, so you can get and stay fit. We know this isn't a cinch, which is why you get major points for taking action.

By now, you probably realize that if you really want to get stronger, fitter, healthier, slimmer, and/or sexier, then you're going to have to reach out and grab hold of that brass ring—the one that's attached to moving more often, eating more wholesome foods, and developing a kick-ass mind-set. It's the only way to become the fit, fabulous version of yourself that you were always meant to be.

In the process of strengthening your body and your mind, you have embarked on a journey of self-discovery, one that has undoubtedly started to broaden the way you see yourself. Take pride in who you're becoming; you'll soon discover that your comfort zone will broaden as you continue pushing your limits both in the fitness realm and in life. You'll gain a new, improved view of yourself as a confident, capable woman who can kick butt at the gym or the office, on the field or the court, and in any and all other domains.

Taking care of yourself in this way will enable you to embrace your life more fully. Open yourself up to taking smart risks, and make bolder, better decisions for yourself, ones that will further expand or upgrade your health and well-being. You'll continue to discover what you are truly capable of physically, mentally, emotionally, socially, and professionally—and become more ready, willing, and able to scale new heights in so many areas of your life. In other words, you are in the process of setting a positive chain reaction into motion, one that will improve every facet of your life.

Feel it, believe in it, bask in it, and commit to it. Own the effort you're making to become your strongest, healthiest, sexiest self, and take full possession of your body as you transform it. The process is entirely in your hands, so it's important to make a conscious effort to maintain your focus, energy, determination, and enthusiasm for the body evolution you're going through and the mental fortitude you're developing. Putting the elements described in this book together will allow you to stop living a broken record of bad diet and movement choices and negative thoughts, if those have been issues for you in the past, and replace them with positive actions and a take-charge attitude.

As time goes on, you'll want to tweak the advice and suggestions in this book to make them work for you; use them as the building blocks or stepping-stones that will bring you toward more fulfilling accomplishments. Once you become familiar with the workouts and acclimatized to them, feel free to make little changes that will spark greater benefits—switch the order of the exercises, adjust the amount of weight you're using or the reps you're doing, try new forms of cardio, or change the length of your workouts. Tinkering with your approach at least every six weeks will help you keep your body guessing and shock it fit because you'll be giving your muscles new challenges that will help them develop greater strength and thrive. (*Note:* It's a good idea to do the same thing with your diet and its preparation so you don't end up in a food rut.)

Also, be sure to check in with yourself regularly to update what's motivating you; as you gain strength, fitness, and confidence, your reasons for wanting to take your program to the next level will likely shift. Let them. This will help prevent your routine from becoming stale, static, or otherwise ho-hum, and allow you to continue to reap the feel-good benefits of fitness and ongoing self-discovery. What started out as a desire to feel more comfortable in your body and get healthier may morph into a more competitive spirit, whereby you want to push yourself with challenging races or boot-camp-style workouts to see what you are truly capable of; if you're already doing races or workouts like those, you may feel inspired to crank up your efforts even more or to tackle more arduous challenges (a triathlon, perhaps?). *That's all good!*

The Get-Strong, Stay-Strong Rules for Life

When it comes to getting and staying fit, certain rules apply to just about everyone. Take these maxims to heart and heed them as if they were gospel, and you'll keep yourself on the right course to becoming healthier, happier, more energized, and more productive for life. That's right! You'll enhance the likelihood that you'll get and stay strong and fit for the rest of your life if you live by the following twelve guidelines. Some of them may sound like fortune-cookie wisdom, but if you really think about them and live in sync with them, you'll discover their true value.

1. **MOVE LIKE YOU MEAN IT—WITH PURPOSE!** Don't phone in your efforts. Get your head and body into the game (that is, program) and perform your workouts with the intention of pushing your limits and making the results you want happen.

2. **AIM HIGH BUT STAY REALISTIC.** It's great to continuously reach for the brass ring—so long as you have even a remote prayer of grabbing it. Framing your goals so they're challenging but also attainable will help you avoid frustration and disappointment and stay on course. Be patient and trust the process!

3. **GET INTO THE RIGHT INTENSITY ZONE.** Push yourself with your efforts and regularly check in with yourself to see if you're working hard or hardly working.

4. **NEVER TAKE MORE THAN TWO DAYS OFF IN A ROW.** Consistency is the watchword of progress when it comes to fitness. If you want to reap maximum results and optimal health from the program, you'll need to work out at least five days a week. It's that simple.

5. SEEK VARIETY IN MOVEMENT AND IN LIFE. Doing so will allow you to keep your regimen interesting and fresh and help you avoid injuries and burnout.

6. HOLD YOURSELF ACCOUNTABLE. No one but you can make this transformation happen. So empower yourself with the responsibility of doing so and don't let yourself off the hook with lame excuses. Go public with your goals. Track your efforts to attain them. Schedule your workouts as if they were sacred appointments (they are, really).

7. TREAT YOURSELF LIKE AN ATHLETE. That means carving out ample time for sleep, rest, stress relief, healthy meals, and other (natural) performance-enhancing measures. Given the way you're pushing yourself physically and mentally, you deserve the right support, so make the development of healthy lifestyle habits a priority. And regularly take time to restore, recharge, and refresh your body and mind with activities that replenish your energy reserves.

8. CHOOSE ACTIVITIES YOU LOVE OR FIND WAYS TO LOVE THEM. *Who says exercise needs to feel like work?!* Give yourself an attitude adjustment and view your workouts as a form of play so you can look forward to them. Seek out physical activities that make you feel good or challenge you in all the right ways and embrace the power of (physical) play. After all, most of us are naturally motivated to do things we enjoy.

9. STAY FLEXIBLE IN MIND AND BODY. Stretch your muscles and your mind to prevent stiffness and rigidity from setting in. If a particular approach doesn't work, try another. Developing physical and mental flexibility is essential to becoming hardy, resilient, tenacious, and strong.

10. PAY ATTENTION TO THE FEEL-GOOD PERKS. If you make a point of noticing how your workouts help clear the cobwebs from your mind or how they improve your mood or energy levels, you'll be inspired to keep up the good work.

11. REWARD YOURSELF APPROPRIATELY. Yes, getting fit and strong really do carry their own rewards, but you should also give yourself regular pats on the back or mental high fives to keep on doing what you're doing. And if a well-timed, health-promoting treat (perhaps some new workout gear?) helps rev you up after reaching a major milestone, hey, more power to you!

12. KEEP YOUR SIGHTS ON THE GOLDEN TICKET. Don't get complacent about your efforts or your accomplishments. Keep striving to achieve new personal bests, to push your limits and seek new challenges, to create the absolute best version of yourself.

Continue to inspire yourself and make good choices that allow you to fulfill your potential and become who you want to be, physically, mentally, emotionally, socially, professionally, and spiritually. Remember, you're the one who is in the driver's seat. You're the one wearing the ruby slippers. You've got the power in your feet, your legs, your core, your arms and shoulders—and in your head. So keep putting it to good use!

As you probably recognize by now, developing a strong, powerful body and mind comes from proper planning, a laser focus, consistency, determination, and a full-throttle effort. Give this quest the respect and attention it deserves and you'll never regret it. Take pride in what you're doing because you are truly giving yourself a gift—the gift of boosting your health and energy, the benefits of taking greater charge of your life, and the pleasure of looking, feeling, and functioning at your unadulterated best. *What could be better than that?*

Congratulations—you are now officially unstoppable!

Acknowledgments

We would both like to thank all the badass women we've encountered in our lives who have inspired us to get strong, stay sharp, and pursue our goals with full force. Without them, we wouldn't be where we are today—nor would we have written this book. In addition, we would like to thank our agent, Rick Broadhead, who got behind this project with great enthusiasm and was incredibly supportive from start to finish. We are deeply grateful for the passion, encouragement, and smart editing provided by our editor, Heather Jackson at Crown. Without Heather's brilliant vision for this book, it simply wouldn't have happened; her support and guidance have been invaluable and are much appreciated.

We also want to thank David Kirchhoff, the former CEO of Weight Watchers International, for writing the foreword to this book and the folks at Weight Watchers who brought the two of us together on several editorial projects. A huge shout-out to Leslie Bonci, MPH, RD, director of sports nutrition at the University of Pittsburgh Medical Center and author of *Walk Your Butt Off*, and Tara Gidus, MS, RD, a nutritionist based in Orlando and author of *The Flat Belly Cookbook for Dummies*, for sharing their nutrition wisdom with us.

From Jen: I would like to thank my husband, Noah, for always giving me the freedom to pursue my dreams and for being such a strong believer in me. My constantly active, truly amazing little boy, Dylan, makes me want to be a better person every day and helps me see the really important things in life. I love you more than words can describe! I always need to thank my mom for just being the world's most amazing mother a girl can ask for, today, yesterday, and always, no matter what. I also want to thank my late father, Michael, who gave me a childhood and life I can only hope for every little girl.

From Stacey: I want to thank my extended family and friends for rallying around me on this project and many others. Your support and encouragement mean everything to me. In particular, my deep appreciation goes to my friend Ingrid Martin, who encouraged me to become a certified Spinning instructor and launched my second career (as a fitness professional), something that has truly changed my life. I also want to thank my sons, Nate and Nick, who are my biggest cheerleaders and who inspire me to continue to grow and evolve right along with them.

Exercise Index

General Index

week one foods and meals, 61–63

weeks two and three foods and meals, 63–69

week four and beyond, 69–70

Dinner examples, 63, 67, 69, 70

Drop sets, 193

Dumbbells, for exercises, 82–83. *See also Exercise Index*

E

Eating. *See Diet plan references*

Edamame, 61–62

Eggplant, 64

Eggs, 67, 70

Endive, 62

Endorphins, 22

EPOC (excess postexercise oxygen consumption), 171

Exercises, 191–192

keeping things fresh, 190–193

patterns of (straight sets, super sets, circuit training), 191

rep schemes, 193

specific. *See Exercise Index*

splits (body-part), 190–191

workouts using. *See Workout routines references*

F

Fats, healthy, 59, 67

Fear, facing, 47–50

Fish and seafood, 61, 64, 67, 70

Fitness

assessing. *See Fitness assessment*

commitment to, 30–31

cornerstones of, 21

exercise routines. *See Workout routines references*

exercises for. *See Exercise Index*

healthy eating habits and, 21–22

mental aspect of. *See Mental fitness; Mental strength*

mind-body connection and, 28, 29–30

new 3 Rs for, 22–23

optimizing, 218–220

power grid. *See Workout routines: 4-3-2-1 Power Grid*

smart strategies for, 27

training principles, 24–26

Fitness assessment, 33–38. *See also Lifestyle assessment*

about: overview of, 33

advanced lower-body strength, 37

age of body in fitness years, 42

balance, 38

cardio condition, 33–35

flexibility in hamstrings, lower back, 37–38

lower-body strength, 36

upper-body strength, 35–36

Flexibility

measuring in hamstrings/lower back, 37–38

mental, 51

reforming negative thoughts, 54

stretching for. *See Stretching*

"Flow," being in present moment and, 51

Fluids, 62, 74, 75–76

Food. *See Diet plan references*

Formula, finding, 24

4-3-2-1 Power Grid. *See Workout routines: 4-3-2-1 Power Grid*

Freshness, in workouts, 53

Fruits, 64, 65. *See also specific fruits*

Full-body approach, 190

G

Goals

action-oriented, 24, 45

brag box and, 31

expecting to thrive, 56

realistic, 24, 45

recording progress, 31

relishing your success, 55–56

Goals (*cont.*)
    setting (STAR treatment), 24, 45
    of SINS plan, 14–15
    specific, 24, 45
    storyboard for seeing, 45
    time-based, 24, 45
    tips to achieve. *See* Mental strength
Grains, 58, 61, 64, 66, 68, 73
Grapefruit, 65, 74
Grapes, 65, 69
Greek yogurt. *See* Yogurt
Green beans, 64, 69
Greens, 62
Groin Stretch, 195

H
Habits
    eating. *See Diet plan references*
    energizing, cultivating, 54–55
Hamstring Stretch, 196
Harris-Benedict equation, 71
Heart rate
    cardio condition and, 33–35
    intensity of workouts and,
        214
    monitor for, 83
    taking, 35, 213
    target, calculating, 213
Hemp seeds, 61
Herbs and spices, 62
Higher reps, 193
High-intensity interval training (HIIT).
        See Exercise Index
Hip Flexor Stretch, 196
Hips, measuring, 34
Honeydew melon, 65

I
Inner strength. *See* Mental strength
Inside Sport Psychology (Karageorghis and
        Terry), 46, 54
Intensity, of workouts, 214

J
Jicama, 61

K
Kale, 62
Karageorghis, Costas, 46, 51, 54
Kefir, 61
Kelp, 62
Kiwi, 65
Kleiner, Susan, 74–75

L
Leeks, 64
Legumes. *See* Beans and other
        legumes
Lentils, 61–62
Lettuces, 62
Lifestyle assessment, 38–42. *See also*
        Fitness assessment
    about: overview of, 32–33, 38
    BMI and, 34
    measuring yourself, 34–35
    questions to answer, 39–41
    reasons for, 32–33
    scoring, 41–42
    tools for self-assessment, 34–35
Lower reps, 193
Lunch examples, 62–63, 67, 68, 70

M
Mackerel, 67
Mangoes, 65, 69, 70
Mantra, developing, 46–47
Measurements
    BMI, 34
    bust, 34
    hips, 34
    taking and retaking, 34–35
    value of, 35
    waist, 34
Meats and other proteins, 58, 66–67

Medicine ball, for exercises, 83. *See also Exercise Index*

Melons, 65

Mental fitness
    becoming personal best and, 28–31
    changing internal conversation, 26
    importance of, 26
    mind-body connection and, 28, 29–30
    optimizing, 218–220
    as start of physical fitness, 26
    strengthening mental resolve, 27
    strength of body and, 27–28
    tapping into hidden strengths, 27
    training for, 27
    willpower and, 27–28

Mental strength, 43–56. *See also* Confidence
    being in present, 51
    belief system and, 44
    benefits of, 43, 44–45
    changing mental perception of body and, 43–44
    cultivating energizing habits, 54–55
    expecting to thrive, 56
    facing fears and, 47–50
    fitness mentor and, 52
    focusing on controllable things, 50–51
    handling unexpected challenges, 51
    identifying motivators, 46
    keeping things fresh, 53
    learning from mistakes, 54
    managing moods, 50
    mantra for, 46–47
    mind as ally or enemy, 43
    overcoming slumps, 51–52
    practice, practice, practice, 53–54
    pre-workout rituals, 53
    reclaiming your mind, 43–44
    re-creating winning feeling, 52
    relishing your success, 55–56
    reviewing accomplishments, 53
    self-efficacy and, 44, 54
    setting goals and, 45. *See also* Goals
    strategies for every situation, 48–50
    using negative emotions, 52
    visualizing yourself rocking your performance, 46

Mental tips and tricks
    being in present, 51
    expecting to thrive, 56
    facing fears, 47–50
    fitness mentor for, 52
    focusing on what you can control, 50–51
    keeping things fresh, 53
    managing moods, 50
    measuring intensity of, 214
    overcoming slumps, 51–52
    practice importance, 53–54
    re-creating winning feeling, 52
    refueling after, 74–75. *See also Diet plan references*
    relishing your success, 55–56
    reviewing accomplishments, 53
    rituals before, 53
    strategies for every situation, 48–50
    using negative emotions and, 52

Mentor, fitness, 52

Metabolism
    afterburn effect (EPOC), 171
    breakfast and, 73
    calculating resting rate (RMR), 71–72
    calories and, 70–72, 73, 171
    meal schedule and, 73
    metabolism-boosting foods, 76
    mineral balance and, 74
    revving up, 22, 62, 76, 175, 193, 197–198, 216
    water intake and, 75–76
    water weight and, 74

Mind and behavior. *See* Mental fitness

Minerals. *See* Vitamins and minerals

Mistakes, learning from, 54

Moderate reps, 193

Modified reverse pyramid system. *See also* Workout routines: 4-3-2-1 Power Grid
    afterburn effect (EPOC), 171

circuits pattern (4-3-2-1) explained, 173–174

combining intensity and variety, 171–172

excess postexercise oxygen consumption (EPOC) benefit, 171

as modified reverse pyramid system, 170

pyramid systems and, 169

reverse pyramid systems and, 169–170

warm-up moves, 172

Week 1, 175–179

Week 2, 180–184

Week 3, 180–184

Y

Yogurt, 61, 62, 63, 64, 67, 68, 69, 70, 75

Z

Zucchini, 64, 70